Control
of Migraine

Control
of Migraine

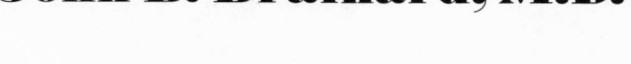

John B. Brainard, M.D.

W·W·NORTON & COMPANY·INC·
NEW YORK

Library of Congress Cataloging in Publication Data
Brainard, John B
        Control of migraine.
        1. Migraine—Prevention.   2. Migraine—Nutritional
aspects.   3. Migraine—Psychosomatic aspects.   I. Title
RC392.B7 1977   616.8′57′05   77–23007
ISBN 0 393 06421 2
                2 3 4 5 6 7 8 9 0

The author gratefully acknowledges the invaluable help of Mrs. Carol Gense in the preparation of the manuscript for this book.

To

Arnulf Ueland,
Vernon D. E. Smith, M.D., and
William F. Hartfiel, M.D.

Who Taught Me So Much

Contents

Introduction

People with severe headaches face a uniquely difficult problem. They may be temporarily totally in-
capacitated by a painful disease process, yet nothing shows on the outside, or can be measured on
the inside. This leads to migraine sufferers being
told that they deserve no sympathy, are just driving themselves too hard, are malingering, have
headaches because they are married (or unmar-
ried), are using their headaches just as an excuse to
avoid social commitments or other responsibilities,
are lazy, or are plain crazy. Sufferers have gone to
many different doctors and clinics without finding
relief, have taken tranquilizers, pain pills, tried
physical therapy, biofeedback, and yoga; tragi-
cally, many have given up, lost hope, or become
hopelessly addicted to drugs. Some have developed a crippling sense of guilt, feeling that the
headaches are somehow their own fault, and that
they are constantly letting their families and
friends down.

The purpose of this book is to help migraine
sufferers realize that they can lead normal lives in

their chosen careers, that there are scientifically proven causes of migraine, and that application of available knowledge will result in the avoidance of most headaches.

Part One

Understanding Migraine

CHAPTER 1

Introduction to Migraine

If you have migraine, it means that you have a vascular (blood circulatory) system sensitive to the migraine process, and you might as well learn to live with it. Occasionally, people suffer from migraine for a short time, usually due to a severe illness, and then recover and never have another headache. But, most victims are born with susceptible arteries and have them for life. This may not be all bad, because migraine sufferers tend to have low blood pressure, which is associated with long life; also, there is the comforting fact that old age tends to make the arteries stiffer and less sensitive, so that migraine headaches seem to disappear with advancing years.

Once you know that you have a migraine-prone vascular system, you have to learn to accept the fact that, when conditions are right, it takes an extremely small amount of a trigger chemical to set off a headache. It is hard to believe that at a party the guest next to you can pour down glass after glass of wine and get nothing but a glow, but if you drink as much as a thimbleful you will be a vegetable the next day. But that's the way it is.

Migraine is the reaction of the human vascular system to certain stimuli. Scientifically, the typical migraine attack involves a severe frontal headache which lasts from a few minutes to as much as forty-eight hours and is accompanied by sensitivity to light, smell, and noise; and by nausea and vomiting, stuffy nose, running eyes, and a feeling of abject misery.

Subjectively, a migraine starts with a dread feeling that it is coming on. You become aware of the fiend inside your head, or you wake in the night and know it is there, lurking in the darkness. You smell something like the filter of a burning cigarette, yet no one is smoking. Then come the lights. There are little sparklers here and there if it's a mild attack, and jagged rings of flashing silver like flickering Northern Lights around your eyes if it's a bad one. Then the ache starts to grow. Your vision becomes distorted; you see people with one eye set higher than the other, or with their noses out of place. You have to walk holding on to the wall to keep from falling. The ache grows around your eye. Your eye waters, your nose becomes stuffed on that side, the ache starts boring deeper. A sudden noise is like a blow on the head. Sunlight is unbearable, people are all shouting, the smell of auto exhaust causes waves of nausea. The ache becomes an intolerable, overwhelming force, driving you to bed, away from people, away from the world, away from everything except the hideous pain which is inside your head.

With fumbling fingers you put some ice cubes in a washrag on your head. "Why can't they be quiet out there?" No one knows how bad a migraine is who has not had the experience. You breathe in gasping sobs. Then, waves of nausea pour over you, and you retch. The foul vomit plugs your nose, the retching shakes your head and worsens the agony. Finally, only bitter bile comes up and you lie back, but the horrible ache is still in your head. Some fool slams a door—if you had the strength you'd kill him. And it goes on, until you ask, "Why doesn't it stop?" and, "Why do I have to bear this?"

Afterward, your hair hurts. You can't comb it, can't bear to lie down and touch your head to the bed. The ache doesn't go away, just tapers off. You can finally keep water down, then orange juice. But you are so feeble, that it's an effort merely to stay alive and do routine things! The lucky ones who never get migraine think you are a weakling and say, "What's the matter with you?" You don't say anything. You think you don't care anymore, you are so engrossed in getting over it. But you do care, and you never forget the mean ones.

You don't sleep well that night. The world looks different for forty-eight hours. Finally, if you're lucky, the fiend is gone and you forget it for a while and pick up your life again.

This condition affects millions of Americans and causes an unbelievable amount of suffering (unbelievable only to those who have never had a migraine attack).

How did I, a surgeon, become involved in treatment of migraine, a "neurological" disease? Simply because I used to suffer from the headaches myself.

So, the system of migraine control presented in this book is the result of personal trial and error, scientific study, experimentation, survey of the medical literature, and testing in my own life and in my patients' lives.

Not all headaches are migraine; the following discussion presupposes that the individual has been diagnosed by a medical doctor as having migraine, and that the numerous other causes of pain in and around the head have been ruled out.

The first migraine in a person's life usually comes like a bolt out of the blue. He or she is probably in the early teens, perfectly healthy, and vigorously active when suddenly knocked flat by a pounding headache over one eye, perhaps preceded by seeing flashing silvery lights. Usually the victim vomits, feels very bad, but recovers in a few hours, perhaps after a short nap. The whole episode may be ascribed to the "flu" by the patient, and may indeed have been precipitated by a viral infection. There may be repeated attacks over the next few months and years, or no more attacks for several years.

As the individual becomes older, the attacks begin to recur at varying intervals—sometimes once a week, sometimes once a month, sometimes almost daily. There may be long free periods when no attacks occur; but when the mature individual is swept into the continuous mill of competitive adult life, migraine becomes a frequent and often crippling influence.

My studies have led to the conclusion that the usual migraine occurs when the stage is set by fatigue (either physical, mental or emotional), and the patient is then subjected to trigger factors which precipitate the attack.

The attack may occur within seconds after exposure to the trigger. Unfortunately, the attack may occur twelve to eighteen hours after exposure. *This is a very important concept, and failure to understand it has prevented many people from realizing that they are recurrently causing their own misery.*

The trigger factors are numerous, and the individual's response to them is quite variable. Each individual with migraine must determine which factors are important to him or her and avoid them religiously. The major trigger factors are:

1. Sudden salt load;
2. Chemical compounds;
3. Foods such as milk, chocolate, nuts, wheat, and pork, among others;
4. Allergies;
5. Physical factors such as altitude, bright or flashing lights, poor circulation of air;
6. Infections.

Each of these factors will be discussed, along with the corresponding stage-setting mechanism. As the discussion progresses, it should become apparent to the migraine sufferer that many common foods, drinks, and conditions previously thought harmless do, in fact, cause or intensify headaches.

CHAPTER 2

Body Changes in Migraine

Before discussing the causes of migraine, it is important to understand what happens medically to the individual undergoing an attack.

When a migraine begins, the blood vessels of the head constrict. During this phase, blood flow to the brain is reduced; and symptoms such as seeing flashing silvery "sparklers" in front of the eyes are produced. The individual may experience behavorial changes, and become hyperactive or short-tempered. This *vasoconstriction* phase (narrowed blood vessels) may last from a few minutes to several hours, and is followed by a phase of *vasodilation,* or opened blood vessels.

Vasodilation is one of the causes of pain in migraine. The pain is usually felt in the forehead, in and behind the eye, on one side of the head. It may be felt on both sides, however, and may involve the entire head. Stretched blood-vessel walls hurt. The individual may also feel the pressure of the heart beating; this causes the throbbing pain. If vasodilation persists, the blood vessel begins to leak, and a complex poly-saccharide chemical moves through the wall of the vessel into the surrounding brain tissue, causing extreme irritation and pain. The head-ache will persist until the body defenses remove or neutralize this chemical. Nausea, vomiting, weakness and severe malaise usually occur with the phase of vasodilation.

Surprisingly, very little is known about the internal control of the migraine process. However, once the process is set off, it seems to follow an inexorable course unless terminated by medical therapy, which will be discussed in Chapter Eight. The migraine may follow the triggering event by only a few minutes, but more often it develops over several hours. Many migraines are triggered in the evening, awaken the victim in the night, and proceed to the most painful phase during the next day or two.

The final phase is recovery. As migraine suff-erers know, you are not quite yourself for at least twenty-four hours after an attack, particularly where vomiting is involved. The recovery phase is usually heralded by the excretion of a large amount of dilute (pale) urine. Migraine patients greet this phenomenon happily, knowing that relief is at hand. As with the acute phase, the body mechanisms of the recovery phase are not known, but adrenal hormone levels may play a part.

CHAPTER 3

Setting the Stage

It is a common observation with migraine sufferers that they tend to get more headaches when they are tired; and yet, they don't get a migraine every time they are tired. Why is this? What does it mean to be "tired"?

Medical science has as yet no precise definition of the term "tired"; so, the best that we can do now is piece together available information to give us a working theory of human fatigue. Apparently, *food and sleep are the vital factors in understanding this phenomenon.* Assuming that the individual has an adequately nutritional daily diet, there is one striking measurable change in human body chemistry that correlates with sleep, the daily variation of adrenal hormone secretion. With about eight hours of sleep at night, the level of circulating adrenal hormone (cortisol) in our bodies is lowest in the wee small hours of the night, then increases toward eight o'clock in the morning, reaches a maximum during the day, and tapers off in the evening. Urinary studies have shown a remarkably similar pattern in the excretion of catecholamines (epinephrine and norepinephrine). All of these chemicals are part of the twenty-four-hour rhythm which regulates body processes on a cyclical basis, and one of their functions is to maintain vascular tone, that is, to prevent *vasodilation*. It seems that with lowered levels of adrenal hormones, the blood vessels are not as well protected against dilation. Thus, while a given dose of a chemical vasodilator will not cause vasodilation in the morning, when adequate levels of adrenal hormone are present, the same dose of the same chemical *will* cause vasodilation—and migraine—in the evening, when the adrenal hormone levels are low.

Translated to the usual migraine patient situation, this means that the victim is more susceptible to attack at any time when his or her adrenal hormone levels may be low. It is known that the adrenals can become depleted by prolonged stress, such as surgery, to the point where replacement must occur or the patient will die. Thus, varying degrees of adrenal depletion may occur with lowered circulating cortisol levels. The "let-down" feeling after a strenuous week of work may reflect this. If a trigger factor is added, the migraine patient then gets the familiar "weekend" headache.

What has all this to do with fatigue? Adrenal hormones may be what make us feel rested or tired. Chemically, the body makes adrenal hormones, stores them in the adrenal gland, and releases them into the circulation according to the demands of stress. If the demand is greater than the supply, the individual may be temporarily adrenal-depleted, and the stage is set for migraine. It seems to make little difference if the stress is physical, emotional or mental; one can feel just as tired after a strenuous mountain climb, an argument with one's spouse, or a college examination. The stress and adrenal drain may be cumulative, gradually allowing demand to overcome supply. (I know of one patient who worked like a house afire from Monday until Thursday, when he would regularly collapse with a migraine. Then, after a weekend's rest, he would be ready to go again, until the next Thursday.)

As will be discussed later, certain factors can cause migraine regardless of the state of fatigue of the individual. Still, in the usual situation, adrenal depletion can set the stage so that a surprisingly small amount of a trigger factor will precipitate a migraine. In the following chapters, we shall explore the trigger factors.

CHAPTER 4

Sudden Salt Load

Many migraine sufferers have found that certain foods "make their headaches worse" and, therefore, they avoid these foods. Many foods and drinks are well-documented trigger factors, and will be discussed later. But there is one factor that does not seem to be generally known, which has proven most significant in migraine control in me and in my patients. That factor is the effect of a sudden salt (sodium chloride) load on the vascular system.

One day during the years when I was being racked with migraines and was searching desperately for relief, I tried taking several salt tablets in the afternoon. The rationale for this was the well-known ability of the sodium ion in the blood stream to exert a marked effect on blood pressure and volume. I reasoned that if the blood vessels could be kept dilated by a sodium load, there would be no vasoconstriction phase and no migraine. How wrong I was! The resulting headache knocked me flat for twenty-four hours; needless to say, I have not taken salt tablets since.

The next discovery was that sodium restriction prevented migraine if other factors were controlled. This came to me unexpectedly, on a high mountain trail, when my wife and I and three other couples were back-packing in the Rockies. The first day out, one of the men developed flu and became weak. Starting at 7,000 feet, we were climbing about 2,000 feet to the night's campsite, which was quite high for ill-conditioned, middle-aged adults used to living at 700 feet. I mention this because the low oxygen content of the air at high altitudes is a potent trigger factor for migraine, as is the exertion of mountain climbing. When my friend weakened, I carried his pack of about 60 pounds up the last 1,000 feet, after taking up my own pack and coming back down. I was plenty tired after we had camped and had our evening snort of vodka. I went to bed early, expecting the worst; but when I woke, I had no migraine! It was several weeks before I figured out why the exertion that ordinarily would have caused a pounding headache had not produced one: back at base camp, still in the mountains, I had got my almost daily headache, which required medication. What was different about the routine at the two camps? It eventually dawned on me that some of the "necessities" of social life that just aren't carried on back-pack trips are hors d'o-euvres. And what are most hors d'oeuvres? Highly salted potato chips, crackers, nuts, and so on. When do you eat them? At the end of the day, during the "happy hour" before dinner, on an empty stomach when you are most tired. Could the amount of sodium in a handful or two of crackers be a trigger factor for migraine? The answer was yes.

Eliminating hors d'oeuvres (and all highly salted snacks) from my diet brought about a dramatic drop in the frequency of my migraine. I was already avoiding the other trigger factors which had proved dangerous to me.

Experience with my patients soon showed that I was not the only one affected by a sudden salt load. It became apparent that salt in cooked food does not seem to cause trouble, presumably because it is mixed and diluted, and because it is slowly emptied from the stomach into the small intestine. However, one exception to this is ham. Many people get headaches from ham, and I believe this is so because it is treated by injecting sodium chloride into the meat. Allergy to pork may be involved, but the amount of sodium chloride in two slices of ham is certainly enough to precipitate migraine in a susceptible individual.

The importance of sodium chloride in migraine is supported by other information. For example, women tend to get more migraines during their menstrual periods, when their bodies retain salt and water; drug treatment to remove the excess salt and water has been helpful in reducing the number of attacks during this time.

Furthermore, women taking birth-control pills often develop migraine or have an accentuation of a previously existing migraine problem, and birth-control pills are notorious for causing salt retention and swelling.

Removal of excess salt and water, during the diuresis of the recovery phase, supports my theory of the role of sodium load in migraine. But what is most important is that the success of restricting a sudden salt load has been clinically shown to control intractable migraine in patients who avoid other trigger factors.

CHAPTER 5

Chemical Triggers

NITROGLYCERINE

Many chemicals act in the body to cause sudden expansion of the blood vessels, known as *arterial dilation*. One of the most potent is nitroglycerine, which is used to dilate the coronary arteries and relieve the chest pain of angina pectoris. Since it acts throughout the body, it also dilates the arteries of the head, so one of the side effects of nitroglycerine is headache. This is the same nitroglycerine used to make dynamite; and, predictably, one of the problems in the manufacture of dynamite is recurrent headache among the factory workers. Nitroglycerine is typical of the problems with chemicals which are extremely useful in our society but are also an unexpected source of headache misery to susceptible individuals.

ALCOHOL

Alcohol is a vasodilator, so all alcoholic drinks can be troublesome. But it is often the chemicals acting with the alcohol which do far more damage. Good liquor contains "tailings" and "fusel oil" which give it flavor; the latter chemicals are often amines, and are potent migraine producers—more so than the alcohol alone. Most migraine patients can drink vodka (which is pure ethyl alcohol and water) only, and they have to take it slowly, diluted in a tall drink. Concentrated drinks like martinis, tossed down rapidly, are good migraine triggers. The body seems to be able to metabolize alcohol at a certain rate. If more alcohol is taken than can be metabolized, the concentration goes up, and at some point a headache is triggered.

I had one migraine patient who got a headache every time he had a cocktail, until I gave him a prescription for a type of ergotamine tablet. He called it his "drinking pill." He would take one before each drink, and never had a headache after that.

Wine is a particularly potent migraine producer, especially red wine. Wine contains aromatic amines which give it its wonderful flavor; it also contains histamine, a well-known body chemical which causes vasodilation. Some people can drink some brands of wine but not others. The chemical composition, as well as the flavor, of wine probably changes from one type to another and from one grape-growing area to another.

It is impossible to determine the exact composition of all distilled and fermented spirits, so not much information is available on their chemical "contaminants" which may cause headaches. Suffice it to say that the more "flavor" an alcoholic drink has, the more likely it is to cause a headache.

On the basis of personal experience with liquor, I would rate brandy the worst headache producer, then wine, then bourbon, then gin, then Scotch, and least of all vodka. All liqueurs should be avoided.

Given the superficial similarities between a migraine attack and a hangover, it may be relevant to point out that the latter is not a "mini-migraine;" however, the two may be related, based on body metabolism of chemical toxins.

The migraine patient, then, does not have to abstain from alcohol, but should be very careful with his or her drinking habits.

MONOSODIUM GLUTAMATE

Monosodium glutamate is a chemical which is added to various foods to enhance their flavor. By painstakingly testing all the ingredients that went into his favorite Chinese meal, Herbert Schaumberg, M.D., identified monosodium glutamate as the cause of headache in the *"Chinese restaurant*

syndrome." Whether the sodium ion or the glutamate is the trigger is questionable, but many people have found that foods to which monosodium
glutamate has been added cause headaches.

The reaction is probably dose-related, and
varies with different dishes. Clear broths, taken at
the start of a meal on an empty stomach, are potent vehicles for migraine production if they contain much monosodium glutamate. A little of the
chemical in a mixed-vegetable dish eaten toward
the end of a meal may not be so harmful.

Little is known about many food additives, but
I suspect that a lot of them are migraine producers.
It stands to reason that flavoring extracts, which
are chemically similar to tyramine and nitroglycerine, can be vasoactive. This does not mean they are
poisonous or even dangerous, but it does mean
that the migraine patient should be on guard
against them.

TYRAMINE

For many patients, eating cheese causes migraine.
The main reason for this is that cheese contains
tyramine, a vasoactive monoamine. Yellow cheese
contains more tyramine than white cheese and is
thus a more potent headache producer. Tyramine
has been studied carefully, and has been found
capable of inducing headaches when fed to suscep-

tible subjects. This means that cheese, which is a universally favorite food, may be causing a lot more headaches than anyone has suspected.

Consider all the delicious cheese snacks and hors d'oeuvres consumed at cocktail time, when people are tired and hungry after a long working day. Add to that the cheese in salad dressings, in sauces, and in such delightful dishes as lasagne, and you begin to get an idea of how often the well-fed migraine patient is exposed to a potent, proven migraine trigger. In addition, cheese contains a fairly high amount of salt, and many cheese snacks are salted or include salted crackers. One final blow—substantial amounts of tyramine are found in certain wines which, with their histamine content, become doubly potent migraine triggers. Red wines are the worst, but any wine—white, rosé, vintage or new—can cause headaches.

CHAPTER 6

Is Allergy Involved?

The role of allergy in migraine is difficult to define. Before we knew about tyramine, when a patient got a headache after eating cheese we said he was "allergic" to cheese. Now that we know that tyramine in this case works by direct chemical action, we can't say the problem is allergy.

The common denominator of all allergy is histamine release at the local tissue level. Histamine is a vasodilator, which means it expands the blood vessels and it is the vasodilation that results in swelling the nasal mucous membranes in, for example, nasal allergy. So, it is entirely possible that histamine acts to dilate the cerebral blood vessels in allergic migraine. We don't know the exact mechanisms as yet, but, whether "allergic" or "chemical" is the reason, we do know that certain foods cause migraine.

Heading the list is chocolate. Chocolate contains *phenylethylamine,* which, like tyramine, is a monoamine and a vasoactive substance. Migraine patients tend to develop headaches within half an hour after eating chocolate, which suggests a direct chemical action rather than the obscure, slower-acting effect of some other migraine triggers. Chocolate often contains milk and salt, which also contribute to migraine production.

When I was a boy, I couldn't eat chocolate because it caused pimples. So, I looked forward to the day when I would be "grown-up" and able to satisfy a pent-up craving for this delicious treat. But with maturity came migraine, and I soon found that chocolate was deadly for me. Probably, by the time I reach old age, eating chocolate will have become "immoral," and I never will get to enjoy it. Oh, well . . . life goes on without it! This is one of the lessons that migraine patients must learn—that they can enjoy a relatively headache-free life if they will discipline themselves to avoid the triggers.

Next on my list is milk. This includes many good things—ice-cream, whole-milk solids, cheese (as previously noted), whipped cream—besides whole milk, which contains a fair amount of salt and a little tyramine, though not as much as cheese. (However, cooked milk—as in bakery products—doesn't seem to be so harmful. Again, it makes a difference whether or not the milk is taken on an empty stomach.)

I used to drink a "malted" every afternoon, and every night I would have a headache. Beyond that, I don't know why milk is so potent a migraine trigger. Yet, since it is not a universal trigger, patients should test themselves to determine their individual sensitivity.

Nuts are also ubiquitous migraine triggers. All nuts are bad for some people, and all it takes is a few fragments of walnut in a toffee bar or cookie to set off a sensitive vascular system. Cashew nuts and peanuts are also very potent. Coconuts deserve special attention because of the widespread use of shredded coconut in desserts, and because some commercial whipped-cream substitutes are made with coconut oil. Thus, the elegant white topping on a piece of pie can flatten a susceptible migraine patient for the next twenty-four hours.

Fresh and canned pineapple bothers me. It may not be part of the nut family, but it contains something that gives me a headache. It is widely used in salads, fruit bowls, as decoration and flavoring on ham; and the juice is a very popular beverage.

Which brings up the subject of ham and pork in general. Many medical authors place pork high on the list of foods that cause "allergic migraine." There may be something in all pork that provokes migraine, but I have had trouble only with ham, which is unique in that it is "cured" (smoked) and is usually injected with large amounts of sodium chloride. According to information found in many nutrition books, a three-ounce slice of ham contains 837 mg. of sodium chloride; that amount is roughly equivalent to two of the standard salt tablets used to combat salt depletion. Thus the average ham dinner, with one thick slice or two or three thin ones, contains an enormous amount of salt. Even people who ordinarily don't get migraines tend to have headaches after eating too much ham. I think it must be the salt that does it.

Bacon is being investigated because frying it results in the presence of certain nitrites which, aside from causing vasodilation, may be carcinogenic (cancer-producing). However, most of us don't eat enough bacon to get headaches, so it is probably not a critical problem—just something for the migraine patient to be wary of pending further investigation.

Wheat is listed as a common cause of allergic migraine, although I have had no trouble with it and would hate to give up bread, rolls, pancakes, and all the other staples made with wheat flour. There are good wheat substitutes available and, if one develops migraine from wheat, its use can be avoided.

Hypoglycemia is a "big word" often listed as a migraine trigger. It means low blood sugar, and requires discussion as a trigger of unknown action.

Simply going for unusually long periods without eating sets off migraine in susceptible individuals. That is one reason why doctors recommend regular meals along with regular hours of sleep for migraine patients. When you don't eat for a long time, your blood sugar tends to go down, presumably because you have used up the easily available sugar provided by your latest meal. (There are intrinsic body-defense mechanisms which keep the level from going too low; by mobilizing stored fat, the body is able to utilize sugar stored in the liver. This means that a late dinner after a busy day may cause the blood sugar to go low enough to trigger the migraine-production mechanism. Once that has happened, even a large meal doesn't seem to stop the relentless progression to a pounding headache. (Non-migraine people get what they call a "hunger headache," which is relieved merely by eating.)

Picture the poor soul with a sensitive vascular system waiting for his or her hostess to produce a late dinner, trying to fill the void by eating salted peanuts and drinking bourbon cocktails. If the hostess finally serves ham, it would be the crowning blow in generating a stupendous migraine that could last through the next day.

Seasonal problems, such as hay fever, are clearly allergic. I don't have hay fever, but I do have headaches more frequently during the fall season. Spring, when the trees blossom, is also a bad time for me. Although hay fever is a relative thing (everyone is sensitive to ragweed pollen if the air count gets high enough), some people are

exquisitely sensitive and get severely stuffed noses,
red, inflamed eyes, and constricted thoats. Others
just sniff a little. Remember that the final stage of
allergy is release of histamine, a vasodilator, in the
body. For the patient with a sensitive cerebral vascular system, headache predominates over nasal
stuffiness, although the latter is a regular compo-
nent of the migraine attack. Even though they
don't have classical hay fever, most of my patients
report similar findings, such as increased incidence of headaches in the spring and fall.

Infections often set off migraine attacks.
Whether the body responds in an allergic manner
to the offending virus or bacteria, or whether the
organism or its toxins directly affect the adrenal
glands or the vascular system, I am not yet sure; it
could be both, or something else. What is important is knowing that the common cold, for example, can cause vascular instability and precipitate
a headache. Adults are largely immune to most
common viruses, and don't often get a full blown
"cold." After exposure to a virus, they may just feel
a little tired or ornery for a day or two, after which
their system will throw off the cold; but the migraine patient will get a headache. I think this
accounts for many of the attacks that seem to come
out of nowhere; therefore, the advice for migraine
patients is to be very careful when they have any
symptoms of a viral or bacterial infection, to avoid
exercise which will exhaust them, and to be ultra-
spartan about avoiding the trigger factors.

This is as good a place as any to mention smoking. Everyone knows now that cigarette smoking may cause lung cancer, emphysema, heart attacks. But what about migraines? The nicotine in cigarette smoke is a powerful drug which affects the blood vessels; just what it does to those of the head is not known. I can assure you that it doesn't help migraine. When I have "fallen off the wagon" in my long battle with the delicious weed and resumed smoking, my headaches have been worse. Smoking causes a chronic chemical bronchitis and sinusitis, with thickening of the mucous membranes of the nose and sinuses. Whether it is the sinusitis or some effect from the nicotine that aggravates migraine, I don't know; but smoking does seem to cause the attacks to recur more frequently.

CHAPTER 7

Physical Factors

High altitude is a classic physical factor which affects everyone to a certain extent. "Altitude sickness" is a well-known but poorly understood condition which affects many people when they suddenly move from sea-level to the mountains. It causes weakness, dizziness, nausea, and headache, or a combination of these symptoms, which are probably related to lower amounts of oxygen in the air at high altitudes. Most people adjust to the heights in a few days, but the transition period can be particularly difficult for a migraine patient.

I learned about altitude and migraine when I went on a skiing trip one year with a hard-drinking crowd in a private plane. We left the midwest prairie in the early morning, opened the bar shortly after take-off, skied in the highest part of Colorado in the afternoon, and stayed that night in a lodge just below the timberline. Half the group had headaches that night, and those of us with migraine spent the night vomiting. I was sick for two days. On subsequent trips I avoided alcohol, took it easy for the first day or two, swallowed a small dose of ergotamine before take-off, and got along much better.

There are several favorite antidotes for altitude sickness among our group, which is made up mostly of doctors. All the antidotes are either diuretics, which help the body eliminate excess salt and water, or ergotamine derivatives. Another effective measure has been to drive out west over a period of one or two days, and spend a day skiing at lower altitudes before going on to the higher slopes. This allows the body to adjust gradually, and cuts out most of the trouble at 11,000 feet where the powder snow is best.

Another physical situation with underlying chemical determinants arises in a crowded room at any altitude. This causes what I call the "party room headache." Picture a typical cocktail party, with many people jammed into a basement room with poor ventilation. The oxygen level in the air is reduced, and the level of carbon dioxide, a potent vasodilator, increased; hence, the suffocating feeling that many people experience is very real. In a migraine patient, these circumstances can trigger an attack. The same thing can occur in a crowded theater, at PTA meetings, family reunions, in school rooms, or any place where a lot of people are crowded into a poorly ventilated room. This explains why migraine patients learn to avoid such situations. They are not anti-social, as their spouses and friends usually think; they just know that certain social activities will bring on the misery in their heads. The headache brought on by a heated, argumentative PTA meeting is not the result of emotional strain (although strain may help set the stage), but more the result of the carbon dioxide generated at the meeting.

Bright or flickering lights can also cause migraine. I know of one patient who can't drive a car at night because the oncoming headlights of approaching cars rapidly set off a migraine. Most of the time it is not this dramatic, but many of my patients complain of headache after having driven for long distances at night.

I regularly get a headache from watching a color movie on a wide screen, and from outdoor movies where viewing through the windshield further accentuates the flickering light. The only remedy I know for this is to avoid movies or else to take a prophylactic dose of ergotamine before going to the cinema.

One final factor is exposure to sunlight. "Sunburn" reddens the skin because the vessels in the skin are dilated. Whether this vasodilation extends to the cerebral vessels, or whether there is some other effect from ultraviolet light, I don't know;

but it is quite common for patients to develop migraine after basking at the beach and getting an acute sunburn, especially if it is over a large body area. After a tan is acquired, the sun does not seem to cause problems unless the exposure is truly excessive. Consider that sunbathing often includes activities such as beer drinking, eating salty potato chips, salty pretzels, and hot dogs containing nitrites, and it's no wonder that migraine spoils many a vacation.

The fact that migraine can be produced by these physical factors does not mean that the migraine-prone individual has to avoid them entirely. Simple awareness of the problems, and the adoption of a watchful vigilance, will allow him or her to live an active, normal life with a minimum of headache.

CHAPTER 8

Medical
Treatment

Let me reiterate: no one should assume that he or she has vascular headache unless this condition has been diagnosed by a medical doctor, who is the only one qualified to prescribe drug treatment. All drugs are dangerous, particularly those used in the treatment of severe migraine.

Why hasn't the medical profession done more for headache patients? In the first place, victims almost never die from migraine; most people have their headaches, but are apparently perfectly healthy between attacks. Migraine does not seem to be inherently damaging to the patient, so why be too vigorous in treatment?

In the second place, treatment may involve the use of narcotic analgesics, and doctors do not want to make drug addicts out of their patients. This is a very real danger if powerful drugs are given frequently.

In the third place, many doctors think that the headaches will go away if the patient simply avoids "strain"—that is, withdraws from all social contact and stops working. But who can afford to do that?

The usual medical treatment has been for the doctor to advise the patient to avoid as much stress and strain as possible, get adequate rest, plan a reasonable recreation and relaxation program, and take drugs as prescribed for acute attacks.

The drugs used by migraine sufferers fall into four main categories. The first includes non-narcotic pain relievers, principally aspirin, phenacetin, and propoxyphene. These are available in tablets or capsules of the single drug, or in combination with each other and with caffeine. Caffeine is helpful in that it acts to constrict the cerebral blood vessels and to cause a mild diuresis, or fluid excretion, by the kidneys. Most of the time these drugs, plus rest in a darkened room with an ice bag on the head, are adequate.

If stronger treatment is required, the doctor then prescribes one of the forms of ergotamine. It is available in tablets or capsules, alone, or combined with other drugs; it can also be given as a rectal suppository, which is very helpful when the patient is vomiting and cannot take anything orally. Ergotamine derivatives can also be given intravenously and intramuscularly.

Ergotamine is used because of its ability to constrict the arteries in the head as well as elsewhere in the body, and therein lies its danger. Too much ergotamine can cause the fingers and toes to turn blue and cold, and can even precipitate a heart attack or a stroke, simply by causing the arteries to constrict and shut off the blood supply to a part of the body. Yet, in the proper dosage at the proper time, ergotamines can abort a migraine. Remember how the mechanism of migraine works: the blood vessels in the head first constrict and then dilate. If the dilation can be prevented, so can the headache. Ergotamine, given before dilation or early in its course, can stop the process; thus, the patient should be told to take the prescribed dose of ergotamine as soon as the first symptoms of migraine are noted. However, if the migraine has progressed to the phase where polysaccharide has leaked out of the cerebral vessels, ergotamine will be ineffective.

The third class of drugs includes the narcotic analgesics. These are powerful pain relievers, but can only be used occasionally in severe situations, such as with hospitalized patients under strict medical control.

The fourth class includes the migraine preventives. Although many drugs are under intensive investigation for this purpose, only *methysergide* has stood the test of time in migraine prevention. This is a potent drug with serious side effects, but it sometimes works very well. The company that manufactures methysergide states candidly that the drug's method of action is not known; my guess is that it acts by constant mild constriction of blood vessels. It has been implicated in retroperitoneal fibrosis, which is a serious condition of massive scar formation in the back of the abdomen.

There is another problem with drugs, aside from classic addiction to narcotics. People have been known to become habituated to "simple" drugs such as aspirin, phenacetin, and caffeine combinations, sold without prescription in drug stores. Phenacetin taken in large doses has been shown to damage the kidneys. Occasionally, a patient will find that he or she feels better when taking these pills and will take six, eight or ten a day on a regular basis. Once your system becomes used to this, stopping the drugs causes withdrawal symptoms. And—you guessed it—one of the major symptoms is headache. So, taking too many drugs may cause a vicious cycle to develop; the more you take the worse the headache when you quit. Caffeine is the stimulant in coffee and tea, and it does give you a lift; however, vascular headaches can quite frequently be precipitated by caffeine withdrawal. The same thing applies to sleeping pills; it is a great temptation to take a barbiturate, if available, to be sure you get a good night's sleep in preparation for the stresses of tomorrow; but there is evidence that barbiturates tend to use up or neutralize the adrenal chemicals. You may indeed sleep better, but the chemically induced deep sleep may result in vasodilation and set you up for more headaches.

If all this sounds alarming, it should. The toxicity of drugs is one of the reasons that understanding the predisposing factors and trigger mechanisms is so important to migraine prevention. The good news is that there *are* ways to minimize and control headaches, without drugs, that work for a majority of migraine sufferers.

CHAPTER 9

Clinical Study

After realizing that a sudden salt load could precipitate a migraine attack in myself, I proceeded to
test a series of patients to find out if salt load both-
ered other sufferers.

After the miserable attack I had given myself
by taking salt tablets, I didn't dare inflict similar
punishment on my patients; instead, I decided to
ask twelve of them to refrain from salty snacks on
an empty stomach at cocktail time, and to compare the results over the next six months with the
previous six-month period. I listed the other common migraine triggers and asked the patients to
avoid these also. All patients had a medical history
of vascular headache, and all had responded to
ergotamine therapy at various times. (Results were
considered *excellent* if the patient was free from
migraine, *good* if the incidence of headaches was
reduced, and *poor* if no change was noted.)

Response to Salt Restriction by Migraine Patients

CASE	RESPONSE
1	Good
2	Excellent
3	Good
4	Poor
5	Excellent
6	Good
7	Good
8	Poor
9	Good
10	Good
11	Excellent
12	Good

Most of the patients (ten out of twelve) responded favorably. In a few, the results were quite dramatic, with the patients stating that migraine was no longer a problem for them. *It was not determined whether the poor respondents were impervious to sudden salt load, or were simply unable to avoid other known or unknown trigger factors.*

This is obviously not a definitive study. However, it did confirm what had proved to be a very helpful bit of knowledge to me in cutting down on my own migraines. Remember, no one had ever noticed this effect of salt load before. To my knowledge, it was not mentioned in the medical literature until I published this study, so I was dealing with a new medical observation. If it had not helped my patients, I would have abandoned the whole idea and assumed that my reaction to salt was a rare personal idiosyncrasy.

One of the measures of a scientific study is "statistical significance." No attempt has been made to evaluate this particular study because the number of cases is too small; it is hoped, then, that large university health centers, with hundreds of patients and the ability to control conditions, will carry out further studies to determine the statistical significance of sudden salt load as a migraine trigger. In the meantime, my patients and I are quite content to go on preventing headaches by carefully avoiding sudden salt load.

After discovering that sudden salt load could precipitate migraine, I began to keep track of the salt intake and output of my surgical patients who developed headaches after surgery. Interestingly enough, almost every patient with a history of migraine developed a headache after surgery. This should not have been a surprise, because doctors regularly give surgical patients who have just undergone very stressful operations intravenous salt solutions. And the first thing they get to eat after major surgery is a very salty "clear liquid" broth.

I soon found that I could terminate postoperative headache by changing the intravenous infusion to sugar water without salt, and by prescribing a powerful diuretic (a drug which causes rapid excretion of salt and water in the urine). The patients voided large amounts of urine, and the headaches ceased in about thirty minutes.

Why couldn't this diuretic be used to treat common migraine as well? The answer is that diuretics have been used in the treatment of migraine for many years, but they haven't been consistently successful. The reason for this lies in the multiple triggers that set off migraine, and, more importantly, in the body's ability to retain sodium in spite of the most powerful diuretics known.

This calls for an explanation of my theory of the basic mechanism of migraine. Some medical authors claim that exotic and poorly understood hormones, such as serotonin and prostaglandins, cause migraine; yet, there is a well-known, carefully researched and documented mechanism which explains the phenomenon of migraine (to a great extent). This is the *renin-angiotensin II-aldosterone mechanism,* known to be intimately involved with regulation of the body's blood pressure and salt concentration. Briefly stated, the mechanism works as follows:

Renin is released from the kidney when there are changes in the blood pressure or salt concentration. Renin is a chemical which acts on substrates in the plasma and other tissues to cause formation of angiotensin II, the most powerful vasoconstrictor known. Angiotensin II then causes the release of aldosterone from the adrenal glands. Aldosterone acts to cause marked retention of sodium (salt) by the kidneys for twenty-four hours or more.

How does this explain the phenomenon of migraine? The release of renin is probably not felt by the patient; but angiotensin II causes the blood vessels to constrict, and vasoconstriction is what is almost universally believed to cause the sparkling lights and other visual changes, sometimes called "aura," that precede migraine.

Aldosterone causes almost total retention of salt, which leaks from the blood vessels of the brain, causing brain edema (swelling caused by fluid). It is almost universally accepted that chemicals leaking from blood vessels in the brain cause the pain of migraine. I submit that edema, whether in the brain cells or interstitial fluid, is an important cause of headache in migraine. Cerebral edema is well accepted as the cause of headache and vomiting after mechanical head injury. This theory fits the fact that cerebral edema after head injury can sometimes be controlled with high doses of cortisone-like drugs, and that migraine headaches can sometimes be terminated by these same drugs.

Research on migraine is difficult because we cannot see inside the living head. However, the medical literature contains a description of a patient with a defect in the scalp and skull, so that a portion of the surface of the brain was visible. This patient was subject to migraine, and when an attack occurred, the brain was seen to bulge outward through the defect in the skull. When it was over, the bulging disappeared. This certainly suggests increased intracranial pressure and cerebral edema.

All this leads to the question, "Why does the head ache in migraine?" If the chemicals angiotensin II and aldosterone act throughout the body, why don't we have swelling and edema elsewhere? The answer is that we do have swelling in our fingers, toes, and other extremities, and many people notice this as a symptom that accompanies their migraine attacks; but the brain is encased in a box of bone and cannot expand. Therefore, unusual pressures are created in the head, thus causing the awful pain.

Patients often ask why the pain of migraine is usually on only one side of the head. If one accepts the hypothesis that (a) the pain is caused by cerebral edema, that (b) edema fluid is water, that (c) water runs downhill, and that (d) most headaches are brewed at night, then it becomes apparent that the side of the head one lies on will be the painful side. I have personally found this to be true; with a moderate headache, I can roll over in bed and shift the pain to the other side of my head after a while, and my "down" nostril becomes stuffed while the "up" one clears. This certainly indicates fluid shift, but it doesn't seem to apply to a severe migraine, where the forces involved are probably too strong to be overcome by a simple shift of position.

This brings up the subject of moderate headaches. Many people with migraine have frequent mild headaches, sometimes daily, between bouts of severe migraine. I think these are all vascular headaches, probably related to the dose of the trigger mechanism and to the state of rest the individual is enjoying. The renin-angiotensin II-aldosterone mechanism may not be an all-or-nothing phenomenon; a high dose of trigger chemical may bring about maximal release of aldosterone and a terrible migraine, but a low dose may cause a milder reaction with moderate brain edema and mild, or "nagging," headache. Some people who never get migraine may well have recurrent mild vascular headache.

I have measured the sodium excretion in the urine of patients both during and after an acute attack of migraine. I found, as have other investigators, that the patient excretes very little sodium during the attack, even though the amount of urine produced is quite large. This, again, is consistent with the salt-retaining action of aldosterone.

Why, then, migraine? Or, why do some people get migraine while others never have a headache in their lives? We all have the renin-angiotensin II-aldosterone system operating in our bodies. The answer probably lies in individual sensitivity to sudden salt load; the non-migraine individual simply excretes the salt, or perhaps has a mild release of aldosterone, and eventually goes on to develop high blood pressure. To understand the migraine reaction, one has to think back on the time when humans were "uncivilized" hunters. We had evolved from the sea, and our internal environment was similar to salty sea water. But we lived on fresh water and ate only wild natural foods, usually very low in salt. So when we did find salt, as at a "salt lick," our bodies learned to react suddenly and retain what they could get in the way of salt. Consequently, we have evolved the remarkably efficient salt retainer *aldosterone*.

Humans no longer eat unsalted natural foods, and most of us eat ten to twelve times as much salt daily as our bodies require. Yet, according to the vast stretches of evolutionary time, we are but just removed from prehistoric homo sapiens, the animal that had to retain every bit of salt it could get. Therefore, migraine may be no more than the body's unnecessary attempt to retain its salt supply. How, then, do the chemical vasoactive triggers fit into this picture?

It happens that the release of renin by the kidneys depends on blood-pressure changes as well as salt-concentration changes. Vasodilation results in blood pressure fall, which causes the body's efforts to bring the blood pressure back to normal; and one of these mechanisms of increasing blood pressure is activation of angiotensin II and release of aldosterone. Thus, chemical vasodilators may cause headache by almost instant direct action on the cerebral blood vessels (as in nitroglycerine headache), and they may trigger the slower-acting, but longer-lasting, renin-angiotensin II-aldosterone mechanism.

This is a complex hypothesis, but it explains the variation in time with which migraine occurs following the victim's exposure to the different triggers.

With this background of information, how can one go about protecting oneself against the onslaught of migraine in our modern world? Some possible solutions to this problem are discussed in the second part of this book.

Part Two

Living
Without Migraine

CHAPTER 10

See Your Doctor

Now that you have a basic understanding of what I think of the migraine process, how do you go about ridding yourself of migraine?

The first thing to do is to see your doctor. He or she may be a primary physician (general practitioner), internist, neurologist, gynecologist or pediatrician. Tell the doctor your story and find out if you have migraine or vascular headaches. Don't object if the doctor orders a number of blood tests, x-rays, and other tests. The diagnosis of migraine can sometimes be made rapidly by medical history alone, but often numerous tests are necessary in order to rule out other causes of head pain. Remember, you are starting on a life-time program, so the cost of establishing an accurate diagnosis is money well spent. Remember also that there are many conditions, ranging from eye strain to brain tumor, that mimic migraine. The doctor has to consider these possibilities, as well as your general health in planning therapy, especially with drugs. Possible concurrent diseases also come into consideration.

If the medical history, physical examination, and laboratory tests reveal no other cause for your pain, then vascular headache (or migraine) is a presumptive diagnosis. I say "presumptive" because there is nothing that can be biopsied or cultured to prove specifically that you have migraine. The long-term response to treatment is important in finally establishing the diagnosis, so stick with your doctor. You are going to need him (or her) for medication and treatment when you get nailed by an unavoidable migraine (such as from a virus infection), and for general care as well. Migraine does not make you immune to other diseases, and you don't want to fall into the trap of blaming it for everything.

Once the diagnosis of migraine has been established, you have to start avoiding the migraine triggers that were described in Part One of this book. How to do that will be covered in the next few chapters. But while you are learning, your doctor will probably prescribe a drug called *ergotamine.* This should help counteract the inevitable indiscretions (just a small chocolate sundae, for example). As mentioned before, this drug causes

the arteries to constrict, preventing vasodilation
and subsequent headache. Ergotamine can be
given intravenously to stop a severe attack. It can
also be given by intramuscular injection, by inhala-
tor, by rectal suppository, or taken orally in the
form of pills. The latter route is usually the sim-
plest and most convenient, *but leave the method
and the dosage up to your doctor.* There are very
good medical reasons, such as presence of vomiting or concurrent arteriosclerosis, for preferring
one type of ergotamine over another in individual
cases.

Here is a list of known migraine triggers.
There are probably many more, but if you can
avoid the ones on this list, you should notice a vast
difference in the frequency of your headaches.

1. Salt load (a small amount on an empty
   stomach, a moderate amount with meals)
2. Cheese (yellow cheese in particular)
3. Chocolate (including cola drinks)
4. Ham
5. Milk and ice cream (cooked milk is not as
   bad)
6. Monosodium glutamate (bad in anything)
7. Nuts (including coconut and coconut-oil,
   peanuts, walnuts, etc.)
8. Pineapple (especially when fresh)
9. Alcohol:
   Beer

Wine (red wine is the worst, but all wines
    can be triggers)
Bourbon
Scotch
Gin
Liqueurs and brandy (ounce for ounce,
    probably the most potent triggers)

This may seem like an overwhelming list, but
you will rapidly become familiar with the trigger
substances when you know what they can do.

For me, and for some of the patients who
helped with this study, the mere mention of the
words "ham" and "brandy" is a red flag. We get a
headache just thinking about these triggers, and so
it should become with you.

Taking the most potent factors first, it should
be easy for you to avoid chocolate and nuts. Just
don't eat candy bars, chocolate ice cream, cola
drinks, or cookies made with chocolate or nuts.
These are such universal triggers that all migraine
patients should start by totally eliminating them
from their diet. Later, after your headaches are
controlled, you can test yourself easily by eating,
say, a plain chocolate bar at 6:00 P.M. on an empty
stomach. Eat nothing else, and don't drink any
alcohol. For dinner, plan the same kind of meal
that you have been eating when migraine-free. If
you have an attack that night or the next day, you
will know that chocolate is not for you. And, believe me, you won't want it after you have proven
what it does to you.

After chocolate and nuts, the only main categories left are salt, milk products, monosodium glutamate, and alcohol. I think it is best to start by cutting all of these out completely. Salt is obvious on potato chips, pretzels, crackers; you can taste it. The same applies to highly salted ham, bacon, and so on. When you wake up with a headache, instead of counting sheep, think back to what you had before and during dinner the night before. Chances are you will recall something, like a new cheese dip that was so good, you had a dozen potato chips and crackers with it. Then, was it the cheese or the salt? I think salt alone is such a potent trigger that you have to blame the salt. To find out if it was the delicious cheese dip, try it some night (after you have recovered) by eating about the same amount, before dinner, on unsalted crackers (you can get these at grocery stores if you look for them.) Matzohs and unsalted "Saltine"–type crackers are also widely available.

Continue analyzing in this manner until a definite pattern emerges of what you can and cannot tolerate. Remember, you can tolerate more of a given trigger when you are rested—so do most of your testing in the evening.

(One important fact to consider when testing is that many patients are not easily susceptible to migraine for forty-eight hours after an attack. If you are just recovering from one attack, you probably won't want to take the chance of precipitating another one anyway.)

Use all the information you accumulate. For example, if you chance to eat a chocolate candy bar at 10:00 AM, when you are feeling fine, and have a pounding headache by noon, that is just as good evidence as an overnight headache that you cannot handle chocolate.

Soon, you will be instinctively avoiding sudden salt load, chocolate, nuts, yellow cheese, wine, and almost all alcoholic drinks except vodka. And you will be playing detective as I do, trying to find out if there is monosodium glutamate in what you eat. (Thank God it costs money or they would put it in everything!) Seriously, meat dishes, such as tenderloin tips in gravy, may be loaded with monosodium glutamate. If you eat frequently at a certain restaurant, it may be wise to talk with the manager and find out exactly in what dishes they use monosodium glutamate, and plan your meals accordingly.

It may be helpful to write down what you eat, keeping a daily food diary. Then, write down when you have a headache, (noting the time it starts and the duration.) As the number of headache-free days increases, you will know that you are making progress. And, conversely, you can check back and pin-point the foods that cause your headaches.

Soon you will develop the wonderful sense that you are finding the "culprits" that have been bothering you. Sometimes it is only one—what a great relief to have him cornered. Once you have found him, it is a pleasure to deny yourself the next one. When you have tasted success, the rewards far outdistance any unhappiness from dietary denial.

CHAPTER 11

The Daily Grind

After seeing the doctor and establishing the diagnosis of migraine, how do you apply what you have learned to daily living? One of the major factors in most of our lives is work. We spend a high percentage of our waking hours working, and this is what takes much of our energy. Remember, it is fatigue that sets the stage for migraine. So, what can be done to lessen the strain of work? Usually nothing. I think it is often not the strain of work but the strain of extra activities piled on top of work that contributes to migraine.

Most of us cannot do much to change the work we do. The patterns of careers and jobs are determined by ambition, education, opportunity and a host of other factors. The homemaker with three small children, living on a fixed salary, cannot change the pattern of life very much. I can't throw

away the training and experience I have ac-
cumulated and stop being a surgeon because I
have migraine. The trick is to follow one's chosen
profession or career in such a manner as to avoid
migraine. You will notice that this rules out the
need for starting a "new life" or "new career" in
California or Pago Pago. It is not necessary to "get
away from it all;" I think that sort of drastic measure has to be followed only in very rare instances.

I can only write specifically about jobs with
which I am familiar; these include office work,
housework, and the work of medical professionals.
But the same underlying principles apply to all
types of work, so that if your occupation is not
included in these general categories, you can still
get the idea for developing a program of your own.

Office work. This usually has the advantage of
regular hours. Thus, there is a time limit on the
energy requirement of the average day. However,
there are migraine-producing situations in many
offices. Since one may be confined to a relatively
limited indoor space, the factors of ventilation,
heat, light, and noise become critical. One of my
patients worked in a small, stuffy, poorly air-condi-
tioned office, with no windows. With the temperature at 89°F. all the time, and with four typewriters
going constantly, it was no surprise that she had a
headache daily. When she moved to a new office
with good air-conditioning and temperature control, the number of headaches decreased mark-
edly. With enlightened business attitudes towards

employees and with labor unions, "sweat shops" are a thing of the past; but all too often, low-level supervisors are incompetent or sadistic, and building maintenance is poor, allowing for less than ideal conditions to develop and persist. Cramming too many people into a poorly-ventilated office creates the same situation as that which results in "cocktail-party headache"—there is too little oxygen and too much carbon dioxide in the air. So, if you are an office worker, pick a company that provides good basic working conditions. Then, be aware of any physical factors that might precipitate migraine; should they develop, change to another office or start campaigning to improve conditions where you are.

Make good use of your "break" time. If your office is stuffy, don't spend your coffee break sitting in a smoke-filled, crowded "coffee room," drinking diet pop (which contains a great deal of sodium and is itself a migraine producer). If possible, stick your head outdoors for a few minutes, or walk in the halls where the air may be better.

The same thing applies to your lunch hour. What to eat will be covered in subsequent chapters, but try to get a change of scenery, some fresh air, and a little mental distraction. (A sandwich eaten at your desk while you keep on struggling with work is not conducive to good nutrition or migraine prevention.)

Don't forget about black coffee, or tea. Neither is fattening, and the caffeine they contain, aside from giving you a welcome lift, constricts the blood vessels of the brain, while also causing diuresis or expulsion of fluid through the kidneys. It is the most easily available migraine-preventive drug, and it is used in most combination pills for treatment of migraine.

With cola drinks, diet pop, and milk on the migraine trigger list, you can always have coffee. Tea is almost as good, but doesn't contain quite as much caffeine per cup.

Once you have minimized the migraine factors at work, what you do after, or in addition to, an eight-hour job becomes vitally important. Many people have to rush home after work, fix dinner for their families and supervise their children after work, leaving little time for outside activities. Still, most people have other interests, such as church or social activities, bowling, night school, and hobbies. This is where migraine victims pile on the load that will ultimately exhaust them. A good rule to follow is *don't go out two nights in a row.*

Give your system a chance to recover by going to bed early frequently. Once you get committed to attendance at several clubs, organizations, and social groups, sooner or later they are all going to meet on successive nights. Then you are in for trouble. At the same time, Johnny will come down with the mumps, and you will suddenly have to extend your energy beyond its reasonable limits. This does not mean you have to pass up interesting activities, but you do have to take them one at a time. If you join the bowling team this year, and the bridge club wants you as a regular member, tell them to wait until next year, when you can drop the bowling.

Go to bed early Friday night. After a hard week at work, many people think they should "relax" by going out to a party or the theater on Friday night. If you have migraine, the Friday-night blast is probably what will set you up for a "weekend headache." You are already tired from the constant strain of a full week, so why ask for trouble when you can head off an attack by simply resting when the pressure is off? This way, you will be ready for a good time Saturday, Saturday night, and Sunday.

Work in the home. The next category of work is that collection of jobs performed by family-men and-women at home. The pressure, and accompanying acceleration of headaches, usually becomes severe with the arrival of children. Pregnancy, interestingly enough, may temporarily put a stop to migraines. During pregnancy, there are profound changes in a woman's hormone levels. These changes affect salt and water metabolism, and seem to blunt the migraine process. Occasionally, headaches are worse during pregnancy. I have one patient who never had a headache during her first pregnancy, but with her second baby she developed "morning sickness" and "lived on soda crack-

ers." She had constant migraine during this time;
the reason was, I think, that the crackers were
salted and she was repeatedly triggering her attacks with sudden salt load. The same thing happens to people who drink large amounts of diet
pop in an effort to keep their weight down. On an
empty stomach, the sudden salt load of diet pop
may have disastrous results.

A parent with two or three young children is
busy. He or she is often up at night, especially with
infant feeding. There is a never-ending progression of chores—dishes, diapers, laundry, cleaning.
Fortunately, this usually comes at a time when the
parents are young and able to take it. But what if
one of them has migraine anyway? Well, there are
several things that can be done. You can rest when
the baby does—take a nap in the afternoon. And,
you can cut down on outside activities; this is not
the time to be president of the Junior League (unless you are rich and have plenty of "help"). Fortunately, children grow up and parents can get back
in the social swim soon after the youngsters start
school.
    Probably, control of diet is the most important
thing a homemaker can do to avoid migraine. Usually, the homemaker buys the family food and
plans the meals; thus, he or she can easily avoid the
migraine triggers in food. When the children are
fed milk and cheese, the migraine patient can fix

something else. For example, while the children have milk, crackers, or ice cream with their meals, you can have tea or juice, bread, and fruit with yours.

With all the foods I have listed as causing migraine, just what can the migraine patient eat? The answer is almost everything that is good for him or her, provided it hasn't been "enhanced" with monosodium glutamate.

Let's go through a typical day and I will describe what I eat and don't eat, and how I avoid troublesome foods.

Breakfast, for me and for many Americans, starts with orange juice. I think the frozen concentrate juice is one of the great triumphs of modern food technology; it is easily stored in the freezer compartment of a refrigerator, and is universally available. Best of all, it doesn't cause migraine for me and has escaped "chemical additives." I drink it many times throughout the day, in place of pop or milk at "break" time, as a bedtime snack, as a pick-up when I'm tired, even as a mix at cocktail hour.

To get back to breakfast: cereals and milk are forbidden because of my sensitivity to milk. So, I have bacon and eggs, toast, and coffee. Eggs are high in protein and give me staying power for a busy day. I don't think the egg cholesterol content is dangerous—my serum cholesterol is well below

200 mg. percent. Medical opinion, based on atherosclerosis research, holds that it is the total amount of calories one ingests that is the most important factor in controlling serum cholesterol. If one eats too much, one's liver will make cholesterol out of excess calories no matter what their origin. As far as weight control is concerned, there is almost unanimous opinion that a big breakfast is burned up by the activity of the day. So, for weight control, cut down the evening meal. The high-protein egg breakfast keeps my blood sugar up for a much longer period than does a cereal breakfast. And remember, low blood sugar is a migraine trigger.

Midmorning break usually means black coffee and a sweet roll or doughnut. I get these in the doctors' lounge of the hospital; homemakers can prepare their own, and office workers have access to the company cafeteria. We all have to watch for the same pitfalls if we have migraine. Doughnuts are often chocolate-covered; avoid these, and eat the plain ones. Sweet rolls sometimes contain nuts or, more insidiously, shredded coconut; usually, there is at least one safe kind available without nuts. Break time is when the cola drinker gets into trouble. All cola drinks have a chocolate base, and are therefore migraine causers. Clear, non-cola drinks are all right, provided they don't have high sodium content or contain monosodium glutamate. If you don't like coffee or tea, drink orange juice, apple cider, grapefruit juice or tomato juice.

I have a special warning about cookies, another popular break-time snack. All it takes is the chocolate in one chip of a toll-house cookie to give you a headache if you have a sensitive vascular system. Even more deadly, because they are harder to spot, are nut fragments in cookies. Whatever the chemical is that nuts contain, it is so potent that a few fragments in one cookie will precipitate an attack. If you don't believe me, try it some time when you have mastered the other factors of migraine control. But keep the ergotamine handy.

Lunch time brings more chance for exposure to migraine triggers. For example, homemakers, who can pretty well control what's available for lunch, usually don't want to take the time and energy to fix a hot meal for just one person. So, what happens? A great American favorite is the cheese sandwich, usually made with yellow processed cheese, loaded with tyramine, and washed down with a glass of milk or a "Coke". Look out migraine! Another favorite is a bowl of canned soup. If you examine the labels of our most popular brands of soup, they almost invariably contain monosodium glutamate. The amount may be small but it's there, and it produces migraine. Another sad fact is that the universal peanut butter sandwich causes migraine in susceptible individuals.

So what's to eat at home? Well, there are lots of things. I think that it is important to follow a high-protein diet; as mentioned before, protein prevents the blood sugar from diving several hours

after meals. (Again, keep in mind that low blood
sugar precipitates migraine.) The best sources of
protein are meat, fish, and fowl. But don't use ham,
because it has too much salt. If there aren't any
good leftovers from last night's roast or chicken,
open a can of tuna fish. Fish and chicken are ideal,
because they contain little fat to cause overweight,
are not as expensive as some meats, and can usually be found and fixed without migraine-producing chemical additives. Lunch-meat can also be
good, but test each kind to rule out the presence
of nitrites and too much salt. Drink orange juice,
tea, coffee, or water; avoid cola drinks, diet pop,
milk and alcohol.

When you go out for lunch, don't forget the
lowly hamburger. It is usually one of the least expensive items on the menu, contains high-quality
protein, and has no monosodium glutamate. (I eat
so many hamburgers, my daughters call me
"Wimpy.") When you have migraine, you learn
what you can handle and tend to stick to it. Almost
any kind of meat, fish, or fowl is good. If you have
a salad, remember that Roquefort dressing is made
from cheese, so have French dressing; oil-and-
vinegar is also safe. Similarly, au gratin potatoes
are made with cheese, so have a baked potato or
French fries, although the latter are often heavily
salted and may be a problem. They don't seem to
bother me when eaten with a meal, but I wouldn't
touch them on an empty stomach.

For dessert, ice cream and sundaes are *out*.

You can eat sherbet if it is made without milk, and pie is usually available. Be careful of the gooey, white whipped cream substitutes on many desserts; that delicious-looking white stuff is probably made from a coconut-oil base, and the amount on a piece of pie will knock you flat. (Remember the high potency of nuts and nut-oils in producing migraine.)

When preparing dinner at home, it should be easy to avoid migraine-producing foods. But is it? My wife says that my sensitivities make it impossible for her to be a good cook. She can't use all the good flavors she wants, such as chocolate, cheese, rum. She has a point there; many mixtures, such as macaroni and cheese, are *verboten.* But we seem to survive on meat, potatoes, vegetables and salad, and a small amount of cooked milk in food doesn't bother me. Almost anything cooked from scratch is all right as long as it isn't made with chocolate or nuts. Packaged foods can be dangerous—we recently used a commercial rice mixture which was so good I ate two helpings, but it contained monosodium glutamate and ruined my next day.

One special rule for dinner is to eat early. Evening is the most sensitive time for migraine production; it is then that your body defenses are at their lowest. Many people don't take a break or eat during the afternoon. The interval from lunch to dinner may be six to eight hours, and it's a busy time. Remember, once the migraine process is triggered by going too long without eating, even a good meal doesn't stop it. Parents with young children should feed them early—if they don't, the youngsters can make life intolerable. Also, many working people demand an early dinner. If you, the homemaker, feed the children early, then wait for your own meal until your spouse comes home later, have a snack to tide you over. The same principle of early dinner applies when the children are older; a late dinner prolongs the cocktail hour and invites too much drinking.

When the migraine-sensitive homemaker goes out on what may be a rare occasion, what can happen? Well, if you follow the general pattern of going to a restaurant for drinks and dinner, you may either have a pleasant time or get a miserable migraine, depending on what you do. If you start with a cocktail, you've had it, especially if it's a Manhattan. This contains not only bourbon whiskey, but also red wine (which is an even worse migraine trigger.) The only safe liquor is vodka, which is pure alcohol; it is best taken as a tall drink, mixed with tonic or orange juice. Remember, short, concentrated drinks have more migraine potential than tall, dilute ones.

What you choose for dinner is critical, too. If you have gone to a Chinese restaurant, there is no way to avoid a migraine, unless you have a guarantee from the manager that there will be absolutely no monosodium glutamate added to the food. This chemical is used extensively to enhance the flavor of vegetable dishes, which are included in most

Chinese foods. Remember also that soy sauce has a high salt content. All in all, it is better for the migraine patient simply to avoid Chinese restaurants.

If the diner has gone to a standard American restaurant, he or she should stick to the simple foods such as roast beef, steak, lamb, pork, fish, chicken, turkey, and duck. Mixtures and sauces tend to cause headaches (note that many sauces have a milk or cheese base); we have already mentioned salad dressings. Knowing the causes of migraine, the diner can still eat well in a restaurant, even though the wine and after-dinner liqueur will have to be sacrificed. What could be better than a slice of good roast beef, or a well-prepared fillet of sole? And afterward, there's no reason why a migraine-prone individual can't stay for some dancing or see the floor show; but if he or she "makes a night of it," and stays too long in a crowded bar or restaurant, sooner or later there's bound to be a headache as a result of too many people trying to use too little oxygen. (I've yet to see a well-ventilated night club.)

One of the worst headaches I have ever treated was suffered by a homemaker with young children. She went to a neighbor's wedding (the first night out in three weeks), staying out until about 4:00 A.M. She had had only two drinks the whole time, and spent most of the night chatting and dancing. Ostensibly she was rested, because she hadn't had a night out for three weeks; actually, she was exhausted from the outset by crying children, nighttime feedings, and all the other perils of parenthood. She would never drink at home, and didn't realize that what she drank, brandy, was the most potent vasodilator among all drinks. Thus, she was in the classic migraine situation—overtired and ingesting a dangerous migraine trigger. She might also have had a few salted nuts and a dish of ice cream during the evening. It all seemed, and was, so innocent—but it took her two days to stop vomiting and recover from the attack.

The medical professionals. The final job category to be discussed includes the medical professionals. It should be apparent by now that the rules for avoiding migraine apply to everyone, and that I have simply been describing their application to office workers and homemakers. The avoidance of migraine triggers in food is an obvious universal necessity for all migraine patients.

Nurses have a unique factor with which to contend—the problem of rotating day- and nightwork. Hospital patients require attention round-the clock; you can't close a hospital at five PM each day, as you can a factory or an office. Most hospitals rotate their staff nurses through day and evening shifts in an attempt to distribute the load fairly. A nurse may work the day shift for two days, then take a night or two, and then have a day off. What this does is create a very irregular sleep cycle. If the nurse is subject to migraine, a disturbed sleep cycle makes her headaches almost impossible to control. Some hospitals get around this problem by allowing a few nurses to "float"—that is, to work at different stations every day, but work days or nights only. Some operating rooms have enough staff so that the personnel only work nights once every two weeks or so.

As nurses attain seniority, they tend to get jobs as head nurses or supervisors, where they work the day shift only. But nurses caught in the day-to-night rotation of duty are going to have to resign themselves to an occasional migraine, if they have a sensitive vascular system; and they will have to be even more careful to avoid the triggers than the office worker who has regular hours, hence more physical reserves.

Rotating-shift nursing is probably one of the most extreme examples of a job that sets the stage for migraine. But I wouldn't advise anyone to quit the profession because of this; in fact, the whole point of this book is to show you how you can handle such situations. If, after you have trained yourself to avoid the triggers described in the foregoing pages, and you still have frequent attacks, you can consider working in a doctor's office or an industrial clinic, where the hours are regular. There are viable solutions to the problems inherent in almost every job.

CHAPTER 12

Sex and Migraine

There are so many myths and bad jokes about sex
and headaches that a few observations are necessary.

I have never had a patient complain to me
that sexual intercourse precipitated a migraine attack. On the contrary, loving sex can stop a headache. There is no question that sexual excitation
and orgasm are profound physiological events. Sex
researchers tell us that these events result in increased pulse rate, elevated blood pressure, and
skin flushing over the neck and breasts. These
phenomena are vascular responses, and they must
be mediated by hormone release, either from the
adrenals, from the gonads, or both. This release of
cortisone (or cortisone-like hormones) may some-

how block the migraine process and abort the headache. Increased blood pressure usually means the arteries are constricted, while decreased blood pressure usually means vasodilation. So, it seems reasonable that the powerful pressures of orgasm could effect other vascular phenomena in the body.

What about exhaustion brought on by love-making? Surprisingly, in spite of the overwhelming psychic and physical experience of orgasm, the caloric demand is relatively low. The time interval of active intercourse is limited by male physiological response, and most people seem to sleep better afterward. As one charming patient put it, "Good sex is better than any sleeping pill."

Application of this information requires a certain amount of judgment. A retching, vomiting, miserable man or woman in the depths of a migraine attack is not going to be sexually attractive; neither is he or she going to be interested in sex. As in all love-making, kindness and consideration by both partners are essential. The point is that being susceptible to migraine does not mean that one cannot enjoy a satisfactory sex life.

CHAPTER 13

Parties

Parties and social events tend to put the migraine patient on the spot. Here you are participating in something that is not absolutely necessary. Does this mean that you have to give up all outside activities and become a social recluse? Not at all; the secret is to pace yourself.

As explained in Chapter two, you should avoid going out two nights in a row, unless you aren't working and can sleep all day. Remember Friday night—that is the time to go to bed early and get caught-up after a busy week. Plan your social activities for Saturday night; this is when the best parties are usually scheduled, and most of us can rest on Sunday. Suppose you have your regular bowling night on Thursday, and are invited out to what will be very good social events on Friday and Saturday nights. This is where you will have to be firm; if you go both Thursday and Friday, you probably won't be in shape to go Saturday. Pick what you want to do most, or what you are obligated to do, and turn down the other event. If the invitation is for a weekend house-party, get a substitute for bowling Thursday, and stay home then. The pattern should be clear by now—always maintain a little reserve. Don't keep going until you are totally exhausted. If you do, your system, through migraine, is going to knock you flat and force you to rest, often at an inconvenient time.

Why can't knowledge of the migraine triggers protect you at social events? The reason is, it is so darn hard to avoid all the triggers when you are out. You have to eat and drink what your hosts provide. There are so many chemicals added to our food that, unless you control the ordering and preparation, you are going to get stung. Can you imagine asking your host or hostess at a party, "Did you put monosodium glutamate in the soup?"

There are many things that can be done to minimize the risk. At a cocktail party, most people offer you a choice of drinks, and usually have vodka available. So, have a vodka and tonic. If they only serve beer or wine, you have to forego the pleasure of alcohol and pick a soft drink. But be sure it's not "diet" pop or cola.

When the hors d'oeurves are passed, watch out for the potato chips (salted) and cheese dips. Nuts are out, as are cream spreads. Even green olives can be dangerous, because they are often pickled in brine (salt). Shrimp are safe, as are carrot- and celery-sticks, as long as the celery isn't stuffed with cheese. Unfortunately, sometimes there are no snacks you can eat.

At dinner, the same rules apply as in restaurants. Slices of meat, fish, and fowl are safe, as are salads without cheese dressing. There are always rolls or bread and butter. Plain potatoes, rice and vegetables are fine, but beware of the spicy. While most people with migraine can't tolerate red wine, some can drink a little white wine without trouble. You will have to test your own tolerance: if wine doesn't bother you, enjoy it; if it does, don't weaken—avoid it altogether. Rich desserts are almost always a problem, and here you may quietly abstain. If your hosts notice, they will think you are on a weight-watching diet, which is quite socially acceptable. But don't make a big issue of explaining to them that their prize dessert causes headaches, or you may be responsible for hurt feelings.

Never touch an after-dinner liqueur; all of them are concentrated migraine triggers. This situation is not hopeless, as many people just don't care for liqueurs. Consequently, many hosts will offer you a chance to order a regular drink, and you can have another vodka and tonic. If you don't drink alcohol (and maybe that's not a bad idea), there is no problem. You'll never get a headache from drinking water, unless it's loaded with sodium from a "softening" process.

As long as you are at a party, enjoy yourself.

That's the whole idea of going in the first place. If you are having a good time, the adrenal stimulation that comes from pleasant social interaction will carry you through. Since you have rested the night before, dancing and party games won't precipitate a headache. If you have inadvertently ingested one of the chemical triggers somewhere along the line and get that pre-headache feeling, slip into the bathroom and take some ergotamine.

Most parties end spontaneously at a reasonable time, and you and your spouse should work out ahead of time when to go home. If it's a real humdinger, and looks like it might go on to the wee small hours, think about it a little. If you can rest tomorrow, why not stay? The choice is yours.

A reasonably active social life is good for the migraine patient. Remember that the stage is set for migraine by emotional, as well as physical, exhaustion. (Emotional exhaustion can develop in work situations, where one deals competitively with the same people day after day.) Interaction with other people at social events, bingo games, sports events, etc. can provide a welcome relief to the trapped feeling of the daily grind. Even though they require an energy expenditure, new faces and opinions can give your emotional system a rest, and even give you a new perspective and greater tolerance toward your routine problems.

CHAPTER 14

Travel and Vacations

I remember, from the "bad old days" before I knew about salt load, a skiing trip where I vomited from migraine on the stairway of the airport terminal. (I couldn't make it to the bathroom in time.) Then I sat in misery with an aching head, while we flew to Salt Lake City and drove up to the ski lodge. It took two days before I could start enjoying the trip.

Recently, I flew home from a meeting in Cleveland. The transfer point, Chicago's O'Hare field, was partially closed by a snow–storm. So, we circled the field for several hours, then went back to Cleveland, where I stood in line for an hour to get on another flight, which in turn circled O'Hare for an hour and finally landed. After another hour in line at the ticket window, I got on a flight headed home. The big jets were lined up on the runway, each inhaling the other's exhaust for half an hour before takeoff. I finally made it home ten hours late, having had only two small sandwiches to eat all day, tired, but with no headache.

What made the difference in the two trips? A few years ago I would have been a basket-case after the second trip.

The answers lie in those principles we have been discussing, and show that the migraine patient can maneuver as successfully as anyone in the fume-filled jet age.

The first trip was an evening flight after a very long day, when I had had a ham sandwich and glass of milk for lunch. Furthermore, I had been working very hard, and had been up late the night before, trying to "get everything done" before the trip. So, the first rule is, take time to get caught-up and rested before you leave on a trip. Remember that, once exhaustion has set the stage for migraine, then all it takes is a little extra salt, as in my ham sandwich and milk, to trigger a migraine. If the alternative is spoiling part of your trip (and your family's or friends' trip), it makes sense to plan ahead a little, even to the point of taking a day off to get ready for a major vacation. Then, if you are flying, take a morning flight; pack the day before, get to bed early, and be rested and able to overcome the migraine triggers attendant to air travel.

At the meeting I recently attended in Cleveland, one of the authorities stated that modern commercial jets have the cabin pressure equalized to the atmospheric conditions existing at 7,000 feet. For a sea-coaster or flat-lander, that is like climbing a high mountain; so, the change in oxygen content of the air will be a factor—a migraine trigger. Add to that airline food, which has the usual complement of ham, chocolate, nuts, cheese, and airline drinks (which are usually alcoholic), and you get some idea of the problems to avoid.

On my migraine-free trip from Cleveland, I took an ergotamine tablet as soon as it became apparent that we would have a long, difficult flight. Because of the closed field and disrupted schedules, all we got to eat was a sandwich, fortunately beef and not ham. I turned down the salted nuts. On the final flight, I had another small meat sandwich with coffee. The first flight started in the morning. I had gone to bed early the night before, instead of catching the "last flight out". So, even though I didn't get home until midnight, I made it without a headache.

I remember, also from the "bad old days," an automobile trip where we had to stop at a motel at noon, so I could vomit and suffer with a migraine in bed for the rest of the day.

Now I can drive to Billings or Denver with impunity. How come? Well, on the migrainous trip, I had driven too late the previous night before. (Remember, flashing lights, especially headlights, can be potent triggers.) Then, to keep my strength up while driving, I had liberally ingested salted peanuts, pretzels, potato chips, and whatever else the kids could find in the food basket. And, we had gone through the "frantics," as my children call them, while packing at the last minute, having worked all day instead of taking time off to prepare properly

Now I go to bed early the night before an auto trip. We stop early for lunch, at about 11:00 A.M. or 11:30 A.M. That way, we keep our blood sugar up and miss the crowds at the highway restaurants; we also stop early in the evening. Most of our trips are West and it's tough to face the setting sun as well as the oncoming headlights; so, to avoid further aggravation, I now stop frequently for hamburgers.

To the uninitiated, the maneuvers I have described may seem subtle or inconsequential. To the migraine patient who has had unhappy experiences on the road, these maneuvers can make all the difference in the world. Chances are, your non-migrainous companions won't even notice what you are doing.

I am not an intercontinental traveler, but from what my colleagues tell me, all the precautions needed for domestic travel should be emphasized for foreign travel. Be particularly careful to rest before, and after, trans-oceanic flights across time zones—"jet-lag" is a very real thing. One of my patients tells me it takes at least three days before her system settles down after a flight to Europe.

CHAPTER 15

Age and Migraine

It may be helpful to consider why migraine attacks are more frequent and severe at certain times of life. If one accepts the idea that the stage is set for an attack by stress and exhaustion, why are there periods of relative freedom from migraine at different ages? Unless there is exposure to an overwhelming dose of a chemical trigger (such as nitroglycerine), most patients have few attacks in their late teens and early twenties. Yet, the onset of migraine usually occurs in the early teens.

I think the answer lies in the growth process that takes place from about the ages of twelve to eighteen. During this time, the child is growing rapidly and undergoing the changes of puberty. Many teenagers are frequently tired and weak, in spite of their intermittent frenetic activity, as the growth process alone strains their systems to the utmost. It is, then, reasonable to assume that they will develop periods of relative adrenal insufficiency. If they have a vascular system with a predisposition for migraine, all it would take is a viral infection to precipitate their first attack, and the well-known voracious teenage appetite could account for ingestion of many migraine triggers in food. The uneven pattern of migraine at this age level could be accounted for by the remarkable ability of young people to recover from almost any type of physiological stress.

An interesting fact about migraine patients is that most of them can recall having had "ice-cream tooth pain," or "headache," when they ate ice cream as a teenager or child. People who don't have migraine later in life don't seem to experience this phenomenon as frequently. Whether cold has a specific effect on the cerebral vascular system of a youngster destined to have migraine, I don't know; it's just a bit of information that is helpful in diagnosing the migraine condition.

When an individual reaches the late teens and early twenties, he or she is literally in the prime of life. The body has more ability to withstand stress at this age, and recovers faster from migraine. It is well-known that the best soldiers, from the purely physical standpoint, are young men in the 18–to–25 year age group. Most world records in atheltic competition, such as in the Olympic Games, are set by people in this age group.

There is no doubt that good physical condition improves endurance and the ability to withstand physical stress. For this reason, I strongly recommend a consistent daily exercise program for migraine patients. It is very important to stay in shape at any age; I have found that I have fewer headaches when I am exercising regularly.

Migraine seems to cause the most trouble in the middle years. One no longer has the resilience of early youth, but faces the continuous demands of work, family, and children. A pattern of overwork and chronic fatigue may develop, and, given the standard American way of eating and drinking, the patient is exposed to a constant barrage of migraine triggers. The result is frequent, recurrent and sometimes disabling migraine.

Until medical science figures out some way to desensitize the migraine patient's vascular system, he or she is going to have to be constantly on the watch for hidden migraine triggers.

As arteriosclerosis, which is very widespread, stiffens our arteries, migraine decreases; however, headaches may persist well into the sixties and seventies. Occasionally, migraine will disappear entirely for no apparent reason, which must be delightful for the individual concerned when it occurs.

I would like to close this chapter on an encouraging note. Some of the most active, mentally-alert older people I have known had severe migraine in their middle years. Whether it is the low blood pressure that accompanies vasodilation, or the "governor" effect that migraine-forced rest produces, I don't know; but migraine didn't seem to damage their physical or mental faculties, so maybe it's not *all* bad.

CHAPTER 16

What Not to Eat

The migraine triggers in food may seem to be too numerous to cope with, but they aren't. To help you learn what is safe and what is not, I have listed the common problem foods in groups. The adjacent column suggests substitutes, so you won't starve. Following chapter 18 there is an alphabetical index which will allow you to check a particular item rapidly.

SNACKS

You should *not* eat:	You *can* eat:
Potato chips	Carrots
Popcorn	Celery sticks
Pretzels	Salt-free crackers
Crackers	Hard candy
All nuts, including peanut-butter, coconuts	"Life Savers," "Certs"

You should *not* eat:	You *can* eat:
Olives	Any fresh fruit *except* Pineapple
Cheese	Bread and butter
Cheese dips	Doughnuts
Corn chips	Sweet rolls (without nuts)
Any snack with visible white grains of salt on it or a salty taste	
Chocolate bars	Fruit pies
	Coffee cake (without nuts)
Coconut bars	Most bakery goods (without nuts)
Soft drinks	Coffee, tea, water
Diet pop	
Milk, including skim milk, chocolate milk	Orange juice
Pickled herring	Hard boiled eggs
Dry cereals	Melons

In comparing the two columns, you will notice that all you have to give up is "junk food"—which you shouldn't be eating anyway—and milk products. I have already discussed milk, so you know that you may be able to get away with eating a little, especially when it's cooked.

Cheese. Cheese is a complex problem. There is enough sodium (salt) in cheese to put it on the "forbidden" list if eaten alone or in large quantities. Yet, you may be able to tolerate cooked cheese in such dishes as lasagne, where it is mixed with meat and digested slowly. In addition to salt, yellow cheese (that is, cheddar and processed cheese) also contains tyramine. If it is yellow or orange by virtue of coloring added during processing, it should be avoided. It seems as though the more cheese is handled, processed, packaged, and the more additives it contains, the more migraine-producing it becomes.

What about white cheese, such as the wonderful Roquefort in salad dressing? If it is genuine Roquefort, taken in a small amounts, it is probably all right. But it usually isn't genuine: it is usually "cream Roquefort," to which cream, monosodium glutamate, and Lord–knows–what else has been added.

The complex problems with tyramine in cheese are well illustrated in a study by Kathleen Price and S. E. Smith, published in "The Lancet" (January 15, 1971, page 130). These authors studied the tyramine content of twenty-eight samples of eleven pieces of Gruyère cheese from different sources. They found that the tyramine content of the cheese varied according to the distance from the rind that the sample was taken. Thus, there was much less tyramine present in the center of the cheese than near the rind. The concentration varied from 11 to 1184 micrograms of tyramine per gram of cheese. This enormous variation in tyramine content in one type of cheese could easily account for some patients getting severe reactions to quite small amounts of cheese, while others would get little or no reaction from eating large amounts of the same cheese.

The same investigators measured the absorption of tyramine by the lining of the mouth, and found that significant amounts entered the blood stream as early as five minutes after ingestion. This accounts for the sudden onset of symptoms before digestion, which takes from one-half hour to four hours. It is logical when one considers that nitroglycerine, a vasoactive amine, is routinely given to patients as a tablet to be held under the tongue, where it is absorbed in a few minutes.

As a general rule, the highest levels of tyramine are found in ripened cheese, that is, in cheese where bacterial fermentation is an important part of the manufacturing process, such as camembert. Unripened cheeses, such as cottage cheese, cream cheese, and yogurt, contain barely detectable amounts of tyramine, unless they are allowed to ferment for extended periods.

Aside from tyramine, cheese contains a large amount of sodium, or salt. The highest levels are in pasteurized-process cheese spreads—over seven grams of sodium per pound of cheese. So, a thickly spread sandwich could easily contain enough sodium to precipitate a migraine. Also high in sodium content is Cheddar cheese, commonly called American cheese.

For convenience, I have combined, roughly, the two factors of tyramine and sodium content to rate various cheeses according to their migraine potential. *The worst are at the top of the list, the safest at the bottom:*

Stilton blue
Camembert
Cheddar
Process cheese food
Process cheese spread
Boursault
Emmenthaler
Brick, natural
Gruyère

Mozzarella
Blue
Roquefort
Brie
Parmesan
Roman
Provolone
Gouda
Cottage cheese
Cream cheese

Obviously, the only safe way to avoid trouble is not to eat any cheese at all. And, as stated before, I have found that all other milk products bother me, unless they are cooked. But there is some hope for the confirmed cheese-lover; a center cut of your favorite brand, in small amounts, might be tolerated, in which case you could keep your own supply at home, and just avoid eating cheese when you are out.

Cereals have been included under snacks somewhat arbitrarily. Such things as corn flakes and wheat flakes contain a surprisingly large amount of sodium. The grain itself is low in sodium, but somewhere along the line of manufacturing the flakes, nutrients, puffers, and flavors are added, so that processed dry cereals are very high in sodium, and are therefore potentially migraine-producing. (Cooked cereals, however, are fine.)

SOUPS

You should *not* eat:	You *can* eat:
Chinese soups	Home-made soup
Canned soup	Some cream soups
	Canned diet soup
	(low salt)

This needs a little explaining. I have already pointed out that the problem with Chinese food is the liberal use of monosodium glutamate. If you can find a restaurant that will refrain from using monosodium glutamate, there should be nothing wrong with Chinese soup. The same thing applies to canned soups. Look at the label; they all contain monosodium glutamate. Even if you find some that don't, they are usually highly salted, and therefore should be avoided. Since high-salt foods are a great problem for people with high blood pressure, there are on the market all kinds of canned foods designed for people on low salt diets, so try these. If they don't have monosodium glutamate, they should be all right. Almost all packaged dry soup mixes have monosodium glutamate and are, therefore, migraine-producing. For exceptions, check the labels.

MEAT

You should *not* eat:	You *can* eat:
Ham	Beef
Bacon	Veal
Cold meats (cold cuts)	Lamb
that have nitrite	Chicken
additives	Turkey
Wieners (hot dogs)	Duck
Sausage	Fresh fish
Bologna	
Knockwurst,	
bratwurst, etc.	

It should be readily apparent that you can eat any fresh meat. The problems come when the meat is processed, as in ham, which is literally injected with salt. The meat mixtures, such as cold cuts, are invariably loaded with salt, monosodium glutamate, nitrites for preservatives, or coloring chemicals. For example, a single three-ounce slice of ham contains 837 mg. of sodium. Compare that with a three-ounce slice of beef at 65 mg. of sodium, and you can understand the problem. You feel thirsty after eating ham because the tremendous salt load makes your system demand water to dilute the salt down to the normal blood concentration.

A three-ounce slice of roast pork contains about 60 mg. of sodium. I have had no trouble with roast pork, but many people (as discussed previously in the section dealing with allergies) seem to be allergic to the pork protein itself, and develop headaches via the allergic mechanism. Therefore, all I can say about pork is that you should try it out for yourself. If you don't get a headache after a roast pork dinner, count your blessings and add pork to the list of things you can enjoy.

It is necessary, at this point, to warn you about another trap. Many people have gotten into the horrible habit of rubbing monosodium glutamate on meat before it is cooked. Why anyone would want to spoil a good steak or roast by doing this is beyond me, but they do it. So, if you get nailed by a headache after eating the neighbor's delicious backyard charcoal-grilled steak, don't blame the meat. Many mixtures of flavoring salts sold for the backyard barbecuer contain large amounts of monosodium glutamate, so cook your own steaks or hamburgers with a little old-fashioned plain salt and pepper only.

Be wary of sauces. Tenderloin tips will not cause migraine, but tenderloin tips in savory gravy (as they are usually served) are deadly, because the gravy is "enhanced" with monosodium glutamate. Many of the old stand-by flavorings used to make gravies and sauces contain such things as Worcestershire sauce and soy sauce, both of which are very salty, and may also contain chemical vasodilators.

Vegetables. You can eat all fresh or frozen vegetables. However, canned vegetables can be a problem unless the label says "no salt added." In addition, watch out for monosodium glutamate, especially in mixed vegetables. Who would expect an innocent-looking can of mixed peas, carrots, and corn to give you a headache? The vegetables won't, but the added chemicals will if you eat a large portion. If you're practical, you can usually avoid trouble by simply eating a small portion of canned or mixed vegetables. You *don't* have to give up a second helping of fresh asparagus or tomatoes during the season.

With vegetables, as with meat, watch out for the sauces. Hollandaise sauce contains dry sherry (and a lot of salt). A popular variation contains cultured sour cream, which can be a very potent migraine producer. More than just a taste of either kind sets off headaches with me.

I can't think of anything intrinsically headache-provoking in salads, except the Cheddar cheese slices that are often put in large "chef's salads."

SALADS

You should *not* eat:	You *can* eat:
Roquefort dressing	Oil and vinegar
Thousand Island dressing	Some French dressing
Cream French dressing	Italian dressing
Secret "House" dressings	Mayonnaise

There are so many blends used to make salad dressing that I can't classify them all. It should be obvious that dressings containing cheese, milk, cream, and monosodium glutamate are out. Again, the only way for the individual to know what he or she can tolerate is to experiment. When in doubt while dining out, take oil and vinegar, Italian, or French dressing.

Bear in mind also that salad dressings, even the "safe" ones, are very high in sodium, which apparently comes from the spices and flavors that make dressing what it is. Therefore, you have to use all salad dressing sparingly. This is particularly true when you are dining at a strange table. If you are presented with a salad already dressed with the host's favorite concoction, this is one place where you can eat a little and leave the rest without causing comment. Nobody ever knows whether or not to eat the bottom "holding" lettuce leaves, so salad plates are always left in varying uneaten stages.

DESSERTS

You should *not* eat:	You *can* eat:
Ice cream	Fresh or stewed fruit
Cream pies	Cake without nuts or
Any	chocolate
chocolate-flavored	Fruit pies
dessert	Gelatin
Brownies	Tapioca

You should *not* eat:	You *can* eat:
Any cookies with peanut butter, (including coconut)	Cookies without nuts or chocolate
Whipped cream topping	Jelly roll
White topping made with coconut oil	Pumpkin pie
Egg white desserts	White topping made from soy beans

You should be particularly aware of the high potency of coconut oil topping in producing migraine. There it sits, an innocent-looking little blob of air and sugary white stuff on a piece of pie. But there is something exceedingly irritating to the migrainous vascular system in coconut oil (and in all nut oils), and a few bites of that good-tasting white froth will set you off for forty-eight hours.

ALCOHOLIC DRINKS

The table below is graded by intensity of trigger potential.

You should *not* drink:	You *can* drink:
a. Brandy (avoid all kinds)	a. Vodka
b. Bourbon	b. A little very light Scotch
c. Liqueurs	
d. Heavy Scotch	
e. Rum	
f. Gin	

g. Wine
h. Beer
i. Tequila

The basic problem with liquor is not just the alcohol, but the "tailings" or "fusel oil" which are the by-products of distillation. The body can handle a small amount of pure diluted alcohol, which is what vodka is, but not the complex distillation residues that give various liquors their distinctive flavor. So, light Scotch, which approaches vodka in the amount of contaminants, may be all right for some migraine patients if taken sparingly.

Again, I want to emphasize the migraine potential of diet pop and soft drinks. Only the manufacturers know what is in most of them. As they are taken in liquid form, their chemicals are rapidly absorbed by the intestine, and *Boom!* the headache starts.

Without trying to sound like an organic-food faddist, I would like to point out something that should be obvious from these food lists. The basic natural foods, such as meat, fish, fowl, fruit, vegetables, and most grains are not migraine-provoking. It is only when foods are processed, contain additives, and are flavored and enhanced that they cause headaches. So, when in doubt about whether to eat something, ask yourself, "Is it the basic food, or has it been tampered with?"

CHAPTER 17

How to Handle Crisis Situations

Let's assume you have your work situation and daily life organized, and have identified and learned to avoid substances that really set off your migraines so that you are relatively free of headaches. Suddenly, there is a death in the family and your routine is thrown into a cocked hat. You have to travel, eat out, miss sleep, and spend hours standing around talking to semi-strangers.

This is the time to be very strict in avoiding all the migraine triggers you know affect you. Remember, when you are rested and relaxed, you can tolerate multiple small doses of migraine triggers; but when you are tired, the least little thing will set you off. Also, the stimulation of travel and new surroundings may carry you along for awhile.

The time to watch out is when the pressure is off and you lower your guard.

So, the first rule is *be tough about what you eat.* Don't eat the cheese snacks, wine, nuts and dubious hors d'oeuvres that the airline or Aunt Minnie offers you. You can live on eggs, hamburgers, orange juice and vodka indefinitely.

The second rule is to *eat frequently.* This does not contradict the first rule, because you can get a hamburger or scrambled eggs almost anywhere in this country at almost any time. The point is, don't go for long periods of time without eating, as a drop in the level of blood sugar under a stressful situation will precipitate migraine. If you can't get out to eat, a glass of orange juice and some bread and butter (available in any house) will carry you for a long time. *Don't* resort to eating salted nuts and other snacks.

The third rule is *use your pills judiciously.* If you've had a tough day, and you think you might wake up with a migraine, take one or two ergotamine tablets before going to bed. This is also the time when a non-barbiturate sleeping pill is in order; you are in a strange bed, and need the sleep for a big day tomorrow. You should work out with your doctor beforehand which sleeping pill you can tolerate.

Another difficult situation is the "state" dinner, or meal with the boss or an important client.

If there is a menu to choose from, you will know what to pick. If the menu is limited, remember that with a good slice of beef under your belt, you won't need anything else for hours. If you are simply presented with complex prepared dishes, eat only those you know are safe. If anyone should ask why you don't eat this or that, or if the boss insists you try a favorite gourmet dish, say that you would love to, but you're *allergic* to cheese (or whatever it seems to be made of). Don't say you think it may give you a migraine; most people simply won't understand and will be hurt, or they will think (if they don't know you well) that you are, somehow, "weak." But everyone now knows and understands what "allergic" means, and knows that you can't help it. Chances are that the person you are trying to please may be allergic to, say, laundry soap, has itchy legs, and will be very sympathetic.

Another trying situation arises at sports events —baseball games, football games, and so on. Here, almost everything being sold in the stands is a migraine trigger. Hot dogs have nitrites, peanuts and popcorn are salted, beer has tyramine and other things, and chocolate is unthinkable. One answer I know for this is to prepare yourself beforehand: you are going to be out for a long afternoon at the ball park, so eat a big lunch. The money that other people spend on beer and hot dogs you can spend on a good piece of steak before the game. If you want something to munch on, carry some hard candy in your pocket; and remember, you can always drink black coffee or tea at the game. Another solution is to grab a deli sandwich after lunch and bring it along to an after-work game. If no refrigerator is available, get a roast beef sandwich with no lettuce and no mayonnaise.

A final word on difficult situations; if you are going to the hospital for surgery or for some other reason, don't hesitate to remind your doctor that you have migraine. Tell your physician ahead of time about the specific foods you know set you off, and what medication you usually take for migraine. He or she will be primarily concerned about the gallbladder disease, or whatever it is you are being admitted for, but if you have sounded the alert, your doctor may be able to head off an attack, and can certainly order the proper medication if the nurse reports about your aching head in the middle of the night. Most hospitals have a salt-free or "bland" diet available, and this may be a solution.

CHAPTER 18

It's Up to You

I would like to end this book with a little anecdote about hospitals and soft drinks. A few years ago, when I was the Chief of Surgery at a local hospital, it came to the attention of my Surgery Committee that patients on clear liquid diets were getting liberal amounts of carbonated beverages of the clear variety. To us surgeons, this seemed like an unwise thing to give post-operative patients, because the carbonation of such beverages is caused by carbon dioxide dissolved in cold liquid. When the cold drink is ingested, it is warmed in the stomach to body temperature, causing the carbon dioxide to expand. If the stomach has just been sewn together, the expanding gas could conceivably burst the stitched area open. Carrying the matter a little further, there didn't seem to be any good reason for anyone in a hospital to be drinking "pop". So, we voted to stop allowing carbonated drinks for *all* hospital patients.

The Executive Committee approved our recommendation and carried it out. You should have heard the fuss that was raised! Patients *demanded* their soft drinks—some even cajoled the nurses into running out to the corner store to buy them. The Pediatrics Department screamed that I had taken away one of the few pleasures of sick children; doctors stopped me in the hall and asked what right I had to tell them their patients couldn't have ginger ale. At the next meeting of the Executive Committee the action was revoked, and it ended up with carbonated drinks being kept off the immediate post-surgical diet only. The next day, I saw the soft-drink trucks happily clustered around the receiving dock as before. It was a good lesson to me as to the difficulty of changing people's habits by executive fiat . . . or by doctor's orders.

It is only recently that I have learned of the migraine potential of soft drinks and diet pop. The addictive fervor with which many people consume these drinks was obviously a revelation to me.

But herein lies a crystal-clear example of what this book is about. Such things as soft drinks and diet pop are totally unnecessary for one's survival, and simply by not drinking them you will prevent many migraine headaches.

Other known migraine triggers and determinants have been discussed and explained; the use of this information is up to you.

Appendix A

For easy reference, most commonly used foods are listed and their migraine-producing potential (in individuals with susceptible vascular systems) is estimated.

YES   opposite a food means the migraine patient can eat that particular food with reasonable certainty that it will not give him or her a headache.

NO   opposite a food means the migraine patient should not eat that particular food because it contains a migraine trigger.

MAYBE opposite a food means that the food is not a sure-fire trigger, but sometimes causes trouble in migraine-susceptible individuals. The "maybes" are the ones you have to experiment with, and decide if your particular system is sensitive to them.

ABALONE	YES	BACON,	
ACEROLA	YES	CANADIAN	NO
ALBACORE	YES	BAKING	
ALE	NO	POWDERS	NO
ALEWIFE	YES	BAMBOO	
ALMONDS	NO	SHOOTS (raw)	YES
ANCHOVY	NO	BANANAS	YES
APPLES	YES	BARBECUE	
APPLE		SAUCE	NO
"BROWN		BARLEY	YES
BETTY"	YES	BASS (Black Sea)	YES
APPLE		BASS	
BUTTER	YES	(smallmouth &	
APPLE		largemouth)	YES
JUICE	YES	BASS (striped)	YES
APPLESAUCE	YES	BEANS	
APRICOTS	YES	(common)	MAYBE
ARTICHOKES		BEANS, LIMA	MAYBE
(globe or		BEANS, SNAP	YES
French)	YES	BEANS,	
ASPARAGUS	YES	YELLOW	YES
AVOCADOS		BEEF	YES
(raw)	YES	BEEF,	
		CHIPPED	NO
BABY FOODS	MAYBE	BEEF,	
BACON	NO	CORNED	NO

BEEF, DRIED	NO	BLACKEYE	
BEETS		PEAS	YES
(common, red)	YES	BLUEBERRIES	YES
BEET GREENS		BLANCMANGE	YES
(common)	YES	BLUEFISH	YES
BEVERAGES		BONITO	YES
(alcoholic)		BOSTON	
Beer	NO	BROWN	
Gin, Rum	NO	BREAD	YES
Whisky	NO	BOUILLON	
Wines	NO	(cubes or	
BEVERAGES		powder)	NO
(nonalcoholic)		BOYSEN-	
Carbonated		BERRIES	YES
waters		BRAINS (all	
Sweetened	YES	kinds—beef,	
Unsweet-		calf, hog,	
ened	YES	sheep)	YES
Cola type	NO	BRAN	
Cream sodas	NO	plain	YES
Fruit-flavor		flakes	NO
sodas	NO	BRAZIL NUTS	NO
Ginger ale		BREADS	YES
(pale dry &		BREAD	
golden)	YES	PUDDING	YES
Root beer	YES	BREAD	
Special diet		STICKS	NO
drinks (with		BREAD	
artificial		STUFFING	
sweetener)	NO	MIX	
BISCUIT MIX	MAYBE	(and stuffings	
BLACK-		prepared	
BERRIES	YES	from mix)	MAYBE

BREADFRUIT		Cottage	
(raw)	YES	pudding	
BREAKFAST		(made with	
CEREALS	NO	enriched flour	
BROAD BEANS		& without	
(raw)	MAYBE	sauce)	YES
BROCCOLI	YES	(with	
BROWNIES	NO	chocolate	
BRUSSELS		sauce)	NO
SPROUTS	YES	(with fruit	
BUCKWHEAT		sauce)	YES
PANCAKE		Fruitcake	NO
MIX	YES	Gingerbread	YES
BUFFALOFISH		(plain cake	
(raw)	YES	or cupcake)	YES
BULLHEAD,		(without	
BLACK (raw)	YES	icing)	YES
BURBOT	YES	(with	
BUTTER	YES	chocolate	
BUTTERFISH		icing)	NO
(raw)	YES	(with boiled	
BUTTERMILK	NO	white icing)	YES
BUTTERNUTS	NO	(with	
		uncooked	
CABBAGE	YES	white icing)	YES
CAKES (baked		Pound	
from home		(old-fashioned)	YES
recipes)		Sponge	YES
Angelfood	YES	White	YES
Boston cream		(without	
pie	NO	icing)	YES
Caramel	YES	(with coco-	
Chocolate	NO	nut icing)	NO

(with uncooked white icing)	YES	
Yellow	YES	
(without icing)	YES	
(with caramel icing)	YES	
(with chocolate icing)	NO	
FROZEN, COMMERCIAL, DEVIL'S FOOD	NO	
(with chocolate icing)	NO	
(with whipped-cream filling, chocolate icing)	NO	
CAKE MIXES & CAKES BAKED FROM MIXES		
Angelfood	YES	
Cheesecake	NO	
Chocolate malt	NO	
Coffeecake	YES	
Cupcake	YES	
(cake made with eggs, milk, without icing)	YES	
(cake made with eggs, milk, chocolate icing)	NO	
Devil's food	NO	
Gingerbread	YES	
Honey spice	YES	
Marble	NO	
White	YES	
Yellow	YES	
CAKE ICINGS		
Caramel	YES	
Chocolate	NO	
Coconut	NO	
White	YES	
(uncooked)	YES	
(boiled)	YES	
CAKE ICING MIXES (& icings made from mixes)	NO	
CANDIED FRUITS	YES	

CANDY		CELERY	YES
Butterscotch	YES	CEREALS,	
Candy corn	YES	BREAKFAST	NO
Caramels	NO	CEREVELAT	
Chocolate	NO	(Salami)	MAYBE
Chocolate-		CHARD, SWISS	YES
coated	NO	CHARLOTTE	
Fudge	NO	RUSSE (with	
Gum drops,		ladyfingers,	
starch jelly		whipped-	
pieces	YES	cream	
Hard candy	YES	filling)	NO
Jelly beans	YES	CHEESES,	
Marsh-		NATURAL &	
mallows	YES	PROCESSED;	
Mints,		CHEESE	
uncoated	YES	FOODS,	
Peanut bars	NO	CHEESE	
Peanut brittle	NO	SPREADS	
Sugar-coated	NO	Blue or	
CANTALOUPES	YES	Roquefort	
CARP	YES	type	NO
CARROTS	YES	Brick	NO
CASABA		Camembert	
MELON	YES	(domestic)	NO
CASHEW		Cheddar	
NUTS	NO	(domestic,	
CATFISH		commonly	
(freshwater)	YES	called	
CATSUP	YES	American)	NO
CAULI-		Cottage	MAYBE
FLOWER	YES	Cream	MAYBE
CAVIAR		Limburger	NO
(Sturgeon)	NO	Parmesan	NO

Swiss (domestic) Pasteurized process cheese food, American	NO	CHILI CON CARNE (canned)	MAYBE
		CHILI SAUCE	MAYBE
		CHIVES	YES
	NO	CHOCOLATE (bitter or baking)	NO
Pasteurized process cheese spread, American	NO	CHOP SUEY	MAYBE
		CHOW MEIN	MAYBE
		CIDER	YES
		CLAMS	YES
CHEESE FONDUE (from home recipe)	NO	COCOA & Chocolate-flavored BEVERAGE POWDERS	NO
CHEESE SOUFFLE (from home recipe)	NO	COCOA, DRY POWDER	NO
CHEESE STRAWS	NO	COCONUT CREAM (liquid expressed from grated coconut meat)	NO
CHERRIES	YES		
CHESTNUTS	NO		
CHEWING GUM	YES	COCONUT MEAT	NO
CHICKEN	YES	COCONUT MILK	NO
CHICKPEAS (or garbanzos)	YES	COD	YES
CHICORY, WITLOFF (also called French or Belgian endive)	YES	CODFISH CAKES	YES
		COFFEE (instant, water-soluble solids)	YES

COLA DRINKS	NO	CORN,	
COLESLAW	MAYBE	CANNED	YES
COLLARDS	YES	CORN, FIELD	YES
COOKIES		CORN,	
Assorted,		FROZEN	YES
packaged,		CORN, SWEET	YES
commercial	MAYBE	CORN FLOUR	YES
Brownies with		CORN	
nuts	NO	FRITTERS	YES
Butter, thin,		CORN GRITS	YES
rich	YES	CORN	
Chocolate	NO	MUFFINS	YES
Chocolate		CORN	
chip	NO	PRODUCTS	
Coconut bars	NO	(used mainly	
Fig bars	YES	as	
Gingersnaps	YES	ready-to-eat	
Ladyfingers	YES	breakfast	
Macaroons	NO	cereals)	NO
Marshmallow	YES	CORNBREAD	MAYBE
Molasses	YES	CORN-	
Oatmeal with		STARCH	YES
raisins	YES	COTTONSEED	
Peanut	NO	FLOUR	YES
Raisin	YES	COTTONSEED	
Sandwich-type	NO	OIL	YES
Shortbread	YES	COWPEAS	YES
Sugar (soft,		CRAB	
thick, with		(including	
enriched		blue,	
flour; home		Dungeness,	
recipe)	YES	rock, & king)	YES
Sugar wafers	YES	CRAB,	
Vanilla wafers	YES	CANNED	YES

CRAB,		CRAYFISH	
DEVILED	NO	(fresh-water)	
CRAB		& SPINY	
IMPERIAL	YES	LOBSTER	YES
CRAB-		CREAM,	
APPLES	YES	FLUID	MAYBE
CRACKERS		CREAM SUB-	
Animal	NO	STITUTES,	
Butter	NO	DRIED,	
Cheese	NO	(containing	
Graham	NO	lactose, skim	
(chocolate-		milk, cream	
coated)	NO	& sodium	
(plain)	NO	hexameta-	
(sugar-		phosphate)	MAYBE
honey		CREAM PUFFS	
coated)	NO	(with custard	
Saltines	NO	filling)	MAYBE
Sandwich		CRESS,	
type—		GARDEN	YES
peanut-		CROAKER,	
cheese	NO	ATLANTIC	YES
Soda	NO	CUCUMBERS	YES
Whole-wheat	NO	CUCUMBER	
CRAN-		PICKLES	YES
BERRIES	YES	CURRANTS	YES
CRANBERRY		CUSTARD,	
SAUCE	YES	BAKED	YES
CRANBERRY-			
ORANGE		DANDELION	
RELISH	YES	GREENS	YES
CRAPPIE,		DANISH	
WHITE	YES	PASTRY	YES

DATES	YES	FISH LOAF	YES
DEVILED		FISH STICKS,	
HAM	NO	FROZEN	YES
DOLLY		FLATFISHES	
VARDEN		(flounders,	
TROUT	YES	soles, & sand	
DOUGHNUTS	YES	dabs)	YES
DUCK,		FLOUNDER	YES
DOMESTI-		FRANKFURTERS	NO
CATED	YES	FROG LEGS	YES
DUCK, WILD	YES	FRUIT	
		COCKTAIL	YES
ECLAIRS (with		FRUIT SALAD,	
custard filling		CANNED	YES
& chocolate			
icing)	NO	GARLIC,	
EEL,		CLOVES	YES
AMERICAN	YES	GELATIN	YES
EEL, SMOKED	NO	GIN	NO
EGGS	YES	GINGER ALE	YES
EGGPLANT	YES	GINGERBREAD	YES
		GIZZARD,	
FARINA	YES	CHICKEN	YES
FIGS	YES	GOOSE,	
FILBERTS	NO	DOMESTI-	
FINNAN		CATED	YES
HADDIE,		GOOSEBERRIES	YES
SMOKED	NO	GRAPEFRUIT	YES
FISH CAKES,		GRAPEFRUIT	
COOKED	YES	JUICE &	
FISH FLAKES,		ORANGE	
CANNED	YES	JUICE,	
FISH FLOUR	YES	BLENDED	YES

GRAPEFRUIT		Canned, solids	
PEEL,		& liquid	NO
CANDIED	YES	Pickled,	
GRAPES	YES	Bismarck type	NO
GRAPE JUICE	YES	Salted or	
GROUPER	YES	brined	NO
GUAVAS	YES	Smoked	NO
GUINEA		HICKORY	
HEN	YES	NUTS	NO
		HONEY	YES
HADDOCK	YES	HONEYDEW	
HAKE		MELON	YES
(including		HORSERADISH	YES
Pacific,			
squirrel, &		ICE CREAM &	
silver hake or		FROZEN	
whiting)	YES	CUSTARD	NO
HALIBUT,		ICE CREAM	
ATLANTIC &		CONES	NO
PACIFIC	YES	ICE MILK	NO
HALIBUT,		ICES (water,	
CALIFORNIA	YES	lime)	YES
HALIBUT,		ICINGS &	
GREEN-		ICING	
LAND	YES	MIXES	MAYBE
HAM			
CROQUETTE	NO	JAMS &	
HAMBURGER	YES	PRESERVES	YES
HAZELNUTS	NO	JELLIES	YES
HEADCHEESE	NO		
HEART, ALL		KALE	YES
CLASSES	YES	KIDNEYS (beef,	
HERRING (raw)	YES	hog, lamb)	YES

KINGFISH	YES	LOBSTER	
KNOCKWURST	NO	SALAD	MAYBE
KOHLRABI	YES	LOGAN-	
KUMQUATS	YES	BERRIES	YES
		LOQUATS	YES
LADYFINGERS	YES	LUNCHEON	
LAKE TROUT	YES	MEAT	NO
LAMB	YES		
LARD	YES	MACADAMIA	
LEEKS	YES	NUTS	MAYBE
LEMONS	YES	MACARONI	YES
LEMON JUICE	YES	MACARONI &	
LEMON PEEL	YES	CHEESE	NO
LEMONADE		MACKEREL,	
(frozen)	YES	ATLANTIC	YES
LENTILS	YES	Salted	NO
LETTUCE	YES	Smoked	NO
LIMA BEANS	MAYBE	MALT, DRY	YES
LIMES	YES	MANDARIN	
LIME JUICE	YES	ORANGES	YES
LIMEADE		MANGOS	YES
(frozen)	YES	MARGARINE	YES
LIVER (beef,		MARMALADE,	
calf, chicken,		CITRUS	YES
goose, hog,		MARMALADE	
lamb, turkey)	YES	PLUMS	YES
LIVER		MAYONNAISE	YES
SAUSAGE (or		MEAT LOAF	MAYBE
liverwurst)	MAYBE	MELONS	YES
LOBSTER,		MILK, COW'S	NO
NORTHERN	YES	Fluid	
LOBSTER		(pasteurized	
NEWBURG	MAYBE	& raw)	NO

Skim	NO	NOODLES, CHOW MEIN, CANNED	YES
Evaporated	NO	NUTS	NO
Dry	NO		
Malted	NO	OAT PRODUCTS (used mainly as *hot* breakfast cereals)	YES
Chocolate drink (fluid, commercial)	NO		
Chocolate beverages (homemade)	NO	OAT PRODUCTS (used mainly as *ready-to-eat* breakfast cereals)	NO
Hot chocolate	NO		
MIXED VEGE-TABLES, FROZEN	MAYBE	OCEAN PERCH, ATLANTIC	YES
MOLASSES, CANE	YES	OCEAN PERCH, PACIFIC	YES
MUFFINS, HOME RECIPE	YES	OCTOPUS	YES
MUSHROOMS	YES	OILS	YES
MUSKEL-LUNGE	YES	OKRA	YES
MUSKMELONS	YES	OLEOMAR-GARINE	YES
MUSSELS (Pacific, Atlantic)	YES	OLIVES pickled, canned, or bottled	NO
MUSTARD, PREPARED	YES		
NOODLES, EGG	YES		

OMELET	YES	PASTRY	
ONIONS,		SHELL,	
MATURE	YES	PLAIN	YES
ORANGES	YES	PÂTÉ DE FOIE	
ORANGE		GRAS,	
JUICE	YES	CANNED	YES
ORANGE		PEACHES	YES
PEEL	YES	PEANUTS	NO
ORANGE-		PEANUT	
CRAN-		BUTTERS	NO
BERRY		PEARS	YES
RELISH	YES	PEAS,	
OYSTERS	YES	(edible-pod)	YES
OYSTER STEW	YES	PEAS (green,	
		immature)	YES
PANCAKES,		PECANS	NO
BAKED		PEPPERS,	
FROM		HOT, CHILI	YES
HOME		PEPPERS,	
RECIPE	YES	SWEET,	
PANCAKE &		GARDEN	
WAFFLE		VARIETIES	YES
MIXES	YES	PERCH, WHITE	YES
PANCREAS		PERCH,	
Beef	YES	YELLOW	YES
Calf	YES	PHEASANT	YES
Hog	YES	PICKEREL	YES
PAPAWS	YES	PICKLES	MAYBE
PAPAYAS	YES	PIES (baked pie	
PARSLEY	YES	crust made	
PARSNIPS	YES	with enriched	
PASSION		flour)	
FRUIT	YES	Apple	YES

Banana		PIKE,	
custard	YES	NORTHERN	YES
Blackberry	YES	PIKE,	
Blueberry	YES	WALLEYE	YES
Boston cream	NO	PIMIENTOS,	
Butterscotch	YES	CANNED	
Cherry	YES	(solids &	
Chocolate		liquid)	YES
chiffon	NO	PINEAPPLE	NO
Chocolate		PINEAPPLE	
meringue	NO	JUICE	NO
Coconut		PINE NUTS	NO
custard	NO	PISTACHIO	
Custard	YES	NUTS	NO
Lemon chiffon	YES	PIZZA	MAYBE
Lemon		PLANTAIN	
meringue	YES	(baking	
Mince	YES	banana)	YES
Peach	YES	PLATE	
Pecan	NO	DINNERS	
Pineapple	NO	(frozen,	
Pineapple		commercial)	YES
chiffon	NO	PLUMS	YES
Pineapple		POLLOCK	YES
custard	NO	POMPANO	YES
Pumpkin	YES	POPCORN	NO
Raisin	YES	POPOVERS,	
Rhubarb	YES	BAKED	
Strawberry	YES	FROM	
Sweet potato	YES	HOME	
PIGS' FEET,		RECIPE	YES
PICKLED	NO	PORK, FRESH	MAYBE
PIKE, BLUE	YES	Ham	NO

POTATOES	YES	RADISHES	YES
POTATO		RAISINS	YES
CHIPS	NO	RASPBERRIES	YES
POTATO		RED & GRAY	
SALAD		SNAPPER	YES
FROM		REINDEER	YES
HOME		RENIN	
RECIPE	YES	PRODUCTS	NO
POTATO		RHUBARB	YES
STICKS	NO	RICE	YES
PRETZELS	NO	RICE	
PRICKLY		PRODUCTS	
PEARS	YES	(used mainly	
PRUNES	YES	as hot	
PRUNE JUICE	YES	breakfast	
PRUNE WHIP	YES	cereals)	YES
PUDDINGS		RICE	
WITH		FLAKES	
STARCH		(added	
BASE,		nutrients)	NO
PREPARED		RICE,	
FROM		PUFFED	
HOME		(added	
RECIPE	YES	nutrients	
Chocolate	NO	without salt)	YES
Vanilla	YES	RICE	
PUMPKIN	YES	PUDDING	YES
		ROCKFISH	
QUAIL	YES	(including	
QUINCES	YES	black, canary,	
		yellowtail,	
RABBIT	YES	rasphead, &	
RACCOON	YES	bocaccio)	YES

ROE	YES	SAUSAGE,	
ROLLS &		COLD CUTS,	
BUNS	YES	&	
ROOT BEER	YES	LUNCHEON	
ROSE APPLES	YES	MEATS	NO
RUM	NO	SCALLOPS	YES
RUSK	YES	SCRAPPLE	NO
RUTABAGAS	YES	SEA BASS,	
RYE	YES	WHITE	YES
RYE WAFERS	NO	SEAWEEDS	NO
		SESAME	
SALAD		SEEDS	YES
DRESSINGS,		SHAD	YES
COMMER-		SHERBET,	
CIAL	MAYBE	ORANGE	YES
SALAMI	NO	SHORT-	
SALMON	YES	BREAD	YES
SALT, TABLE	NO	SHRIMP	YES
SALT PORK	NO	SIRUPS	YES
SALT		SMELT,	
STICKS	NO	(Atlantic, Jack	
SAND DAB	YES	& Bay)	YES
SAPOTES		SNAIL	YES
(marmalade		SOFT DRINKS	NO
plums)	YES	SOLE	YES
SARDINES,		SORGHUM	
ATLANTIC,		GRAIN, ALL	
CANNED IN		TYPES	YES
OIL	YES	SOUPS,	
SAUERKRAUT,		CANNED	MAYBE
CANNED		SOUR CREAM	NO
(solids &		SOYBEANS	YES
liquid)	YES	SOY SAUCE	NO

SPAGHETTI	YES	TANGERINES	YES
SPAGHETTI IN		TAPIOCA	YES
TOMATO		TAPIOCA	
SAUCE		DESSERTS	YES
WITH		TAROS	YES
CHEESE	NO	TARTAR	
SPAGHETTI		SAUCE	YES
WITH MEAT		TEA	YES
BALLS IN		THURINGER	NO
TOMATO		TOMATOES,	
SAUCE	YES	RIPE	YES
SPANISH RICE,		TOMATO	
COOKED		CATSUP	YES
FROM		TOMATO	
HOME		CHILI	
RECIPE	YES	SAUCE	YES
SPINACH	YES	TOMATO	
SQUAB	YES	JUICE	YES
SQUASH	YES	TOMATO	
SQUID	YES	JUICE	
STRAWBERRIES	YES	COCKTAIL	YES
STURGEON	YES	TOMATO	
SUCCOTASH	MAYBE	PASTE,	
SUGAR	YES	CANNED	YES
SUNFLOWER		TOMATO	
SEED		PUREE	YES
KERNELS	MAYBE	TONGUE (beef,	
SWEET-		calf, hog,	
BREADS	YES	lamb, sheep)	YES
SWEET		TRIPE, BEEF	YES
POTATOES	YES	TROUT	YES
SWORD-		TUNA	YES
FISH	YES	TUNA SALAD	YES

TURKEY	YES	WHEAT GERM	YES
TURNIPS	YES	WHEAT PRODUCTS (used mainly as *hot* breakfast cereals)	YES
TURNIP GREENS	YES		
VEAL	YES		
VENISON	YES	WHEAT PRODUCTS (used mainly as *ready-to-eat* breakfast cereals)	NO
VIENNA SAUSAGE	NO		
VINEGAR	YES		
VODKA	YES		
WAFFLES	YES	WHISKY	NO
WALNUTS	NO	WHITEFISH, LAKE	YES
WATER CHESTNUTS	MAYBE	WHITE SAUCE	YES
WATER-MELON	YES	WILD RICE	YES
WELSH RAREBIT	NO	WINE	NO
WHEAT, WHOLE GRAIN	YES	YAMS	YES
		YEAST	YES
WHEAT FLOURS	YES	YOGHURT	MAYBE
WHEAT BRAN	YES	ZWIEBACK	YES